DYING TO BE PERFECT

How Teens Can Stay Happy, Healthy and Alive

Robert Michael Cavanaugh, Jr. MD

authorHOUSE®

AuthorHouse™
1663 Liberty Drive
Bloomington, IN 47403
www.authorhouse.com
Phone: 1-800-839-8640

First published by AuthorHouse 10/13/2009

ISBN: 978-1-4490-1522-0 (e)
ISBN: 978-1-4490-1520-6 (sc)
ISBN: 978-1-4490-1521-3 (hc)

Library of Congress Control Number: 2009907991

Printed in the United States of America
Bloomington, Indiana

This book is printed on acid-free paper.

Dedication

This book is dedicated to the memory of my parents, Robert Michael Cavanaugh and Yolanda Sevina Del Monte Cavanaugh, as well as to my beloved wife of 40 years, Marilyn Marie Cavanaugh, and our children, Christina Renee, Andrew Phillip, Teresa Marie, and Nicholas Michael and to all my grandchildren.

CONTENTS

PART THREE

PROLOGUE

Perfect teens can't fly -- they only let themselves down. However, the sky is the limit for those who are happy and healthy, without a care in the world. Even during these complex times, it's still very simple for most teenagers to find a sense of inner peace and tranquility. While adolescents are anything but airheads, they're highly impressionable, and frequently react as if their heart had wings. Unfortunately, this may weaken their ability to resist temptation, and to avoid risky behaviors.

Dying to be Perfect: How Teens Can Stay Happy, Healthy and Alive will serve as a quick reality check for teenagers and parents who are living in a dream world of unrealistic expectations and perfectionist thinking. More than just a survival guide, this book will raise a call to arms for combating the powerful societal pressures that threaten the health and well-being of young people today.

Adolescence is the period of time during which a child becomes an adult. It involves revolutionary physical, mental, and emotional growth and change.

The physical changes of puberty begin with the development of secondary sexual characteristics. In boys these are the growth of facial and pubic hair, and the ability to ejaculate (have an orgasm). In girls they are the growth of breasts and pubic hair, and the beginning of their menstrual cycle (period). Puberty is complete for both boys and girls when they are able to create a child.

It is often not fully appreciated that the brains of young adults are also going through dramatic changes, just like the physical changes in their bodies. As with puberty, the maturing of the adolescent mind can be divided into three stages -- early, middle, and late -- each of which is quite different from the other. Teenagers should not be expected to think like adults until this process of development is complete. It must be expected that adolescents will respond to the pressures of daily living in a unique and personal way, which is highly influenced by the stage of mental growth they have reached.

When children begin adolescence, their minds are usually capable only of *concrete* thinking. This means they think completely in the here and now. For example, those with sensitive skin know that if they stay out in the sun too long they will burn or blister –– they can see it and feel it right away. That's real to them; that's concrete. However, they are unlikely to grasp the concept that sun damage over a period of years may lead to skin cancer; they can't think that far into the future.

Eventually, adolescents grow from concrete thinking to *abstract* thinking. Abstract thinking is the ability to look ahead in a logical way. You can imagine what situations are like, even if you haven't experienced them. Adults are capable of abstract thinking, and achieving it is one of the goals of adolescence. An example of abstract thinking would be the ability to understand the association between excessive sun exposure during adolescence and skin cancer later in life.

Dying to be Perfect: How Teens Can Stay Happy, Healthy and Alive will take you on an imaginary voyage into the mind of the adolescent, and provide unusual insight into what teenagers are thinking, when they are most likely to be thinking it, and why they think the way they do. This book will compare the early, mid, and late stages of adolescent mental growth to the three stages of a space flight, and teach readers how to develop survival skills to overcome social pressures during the launch, orbit, and reentry into adulthood.

The flight plan will include a checklist I created, to help teenagers and their families figure out where they stand, and what to expect with each passing phase. The mission will be to bring the young voyagers back safely, as happy, healthy adults, from their trek into outer space. I have used this scenario in my practice for many years, and have found it to be a very effective way to explain Mother

Nature's expectations as well as modern society's demands for growing up today.

Each chapter of this book is filled with practical suggestions and tips, which follow in order as the story line unfolds. A number of moving, real-life adolescent case histories are also included, to add to the human-interest element of the book. The symbolic journey is written in a humorous tone to discuss serious problems in down-to-earth, everyday language, which teenagers and their parents can easily relate to.

The space flight comparison is very appropriate because adolescents and astronauts share so much in common. This includes the need for keeping open channels of communication and staying connected to the home base as the best chance for completing their mission successfully. They must also be able to take the right safety precautions, to keep the risks and dangers as low as possible.

Adolescents may not be angels from heaven, but they're still too young to take up the harp. While most teenagers are able to escape a close brush with death, each year thousands of American youth are not so lucky. Motor vehicle accidents kill more teenagers than all other causes combined, with 15,000 deaths annually from automobile-related injuries alone. Alcohol and other drugs are known to be factors in many of these fatalities. Many of the 6,000 adolescent murders committed each year also happen when one or both parties are under the influence of drugs or alcohol. Another sobering statistic is that the rate of adolescent suicide has tripled over the past three decades, to 5,000 per year. And it has been estimated that there are 50 to 200 suicide attempts for every death.

Many adolescents also give in to pressures on how to look, feel, and act, as they search for space to grow in a perfectionist society that is obsessed with appearance and the desire for immediate gratification. Every year in this country, one in 10 teenage girls becomes pregnant, and the vast majority of these pregnancies are unplanned. Of the 1 million pregnancies that occur annually in this age group, there are approximately 500,000 live births, 400,000 elective terminations, and 100,000 spontaneous abortions. There are also more than 3 million cases of sexually transmitted diseases, including HIV, reported among adolescents yearly in the United States.

Alcohol use is very common among adolescents, with at least 90% of high school seniors reporting some experience with this drug. Furthermore, 35% of high school seniors have a history of binge drinking, as defined by having five or more drinks at one time, within the two weeks before being interviewed. The use of tobacco and marijuana among youth is an epidemic. Almost 30% of high school seniors say they have smoked cigarettes, and over 20% have gotten high on pot, in the previous month. Of further concern is the fact that alcohol, tobacco, and marijuana are considered gateway drugs, which open the door to use of even more dangerous illicit substances.

As the obsession with being physically thin becomes more important than the desire to be healthy, teenagers often try desperate and even dangerous methods of controlling their weight. To lower their weight, teens often get involved in self-harmful behaviors such as severe caloric deprivation (starvation), the use of diet pills to get rid of natural hunger cravings, and the use of cigarettes or illegal street drugs to control their appetites. They may also engage in different kinds of purging behavior such as making themselves vomit (including the use of emetics to make it easier to throw up), use of laxatives to empty the bowels, or use of diuretics to cause extra urination. Too much exercise to burn off extra calories is another form of purging.

It is estimated that up to 5% of adolescent girls from 15 to 19 years of age have *anorexia nervosa*, a serious eating disorder that is caused by an abnormal fear of being fat. Anorexia leads to poor eating habits that result in malnutrition and excessive weight loss. In addition, at least 10% of college-age females suffer from *bulimia*, a serious eating disorder that involves recurrent episodes of overeating, often followed by the purging behavior described above. While anorexia and bulimia are also seen in male adolescents, girls with eating disorders outnumber boys 10 to one.

As the above statistics show, there is a real need for new efforts to come up with more effective strategies in the field of adolescent preventive services. It is extremely disturbing that these important sources of illness, injury, and death among youth are usually *preventable*.

Teens are often not truly aware of the possibly negative results of their risk-taking behaviors. A strong ability to deny how dangerous a situation is, and a sense that they can do anything and not be hurt, is built right into the mental makeup of adolescents. As a result they are naturally shielded by the belief that "It can't happen to me." But it can, and it *does* happen to them, all in the spirit of exploration and experimentation that has claimed so many victims along the pathway to self-discovery.

As a doctor caring for teenagers for over 30 years, I've had a bird's-eye view of their voyage through adolescence, and I've been in a good position to keep a close eye on the mission, protect open channels of communication, and provide guidance when necessary. My entire career as a physician, educator, and researcher has been dedicated to the care of children, with a special emphasis on the adolescent age group. I'm a board-certified pediatrician with sub-board certification as an adolescent medicine specialist. For the past 28 years I have been the Director of Adolescent Medicine at the SUNY Upstate Medical University in Syracuse. In this capacity, I make a number of yearly presentations at national medical conventions, and have authored numerous articles in the most prestigious pediatric and adolescent journals.

My other career, as a parent, has been shared with Marilyn, the most capable of mothers and my devoted wife of 40 years. Together we have raised four teenagers and witnessed the remarkable changes that occur as a child is transformed into an adult. It is in this role, as a parent, that I have gained an even greater, firsthand appreciation for what adolescence is all about.

Both as a father and a doctor, I have seen the desire to be perfect and the need for immediate gratification demanded by society take a heavy toll on families. I have learned the hard way -- as Doctor Dad -- that it takes a powerful signal to cut through the smog, odor, and pollution of a culture in decay. This book was written so that what I have learned from my rather unusual perspective can serve as a beacon of hope for teens and their parents, as they find their way through puberty's rites of passage.

THE COUNTDOWN

CHAPTER 1
From the Cradle to the Cockpit

As the dawn of puberty arrives, Mother Nature's computers wake the young adolescent up to get ready for the long-anticipated voyage from childhood into the outside world. To use a space flight comparison, years of programming must now be timed properly so the new astronauts will make it safely through the launch, the orbit, and the reentry into adulthood.

As the final countdown begins, the young explorers lie waiting on top of the giant boosters of the spaceship that will blast them into their journey. They are busy going over the flight plan and getting last minute instructions from the adults in mission control.

Checklists, emergency plans, and survival kits are stowed for safekeeping, within easy reach. Every safety preparation anyone can think of has been made. But it's impossible to know every danger ahead of time, and there will be many unexpected challenges.

As the separation from childhood gets closer, the winds of uncertainty often take over, whispering into the crew compartment and flickering alarm lights in the command center. As a result, adolescents and their parents get nervous, not sure they want to go through with it all. An eerie mist or heavy fog may reduce visibility, making everyone even more unsure about what lies ahead. Just when conditions begin to clear up, storm clouds may suddenly gather overhead, casting a shadow of doubt about whether the countdown should continue. Sending up trial balloons to search for safer skies may prove to be a good strategy in such situations, when things don't seem to be going according to plan.

Rather than scrubbing the mission completely, sometimes it may be better to press the hold button and postpone the launch for a while, depending on how strong the confusion is. Before anyone gets too overtired or stressed out, this is a good time to check for any power failures caused by short circuits, blown fuses, or drained batteries. Sometimes only a jump-start is needed for astronauts who are frozen by the fear that they might not perform perfectly from the very beginning. A more complete rewriting of the flight plan may sometimes be needed for those who continue to be paralyzed by the fear of failure.

Family secrets for health and happiness are usually handed down from one generation to the next. However, passing the torch to teens can always be a little tricky. The keepers of the flame must be patient, and be prepared to take some heat. It's easy to get burned when the rockets fire up for a team of rookies in hot pursuit of their lifelong dreams. Unfortunately, happiness may prove to be very hard to find for many young people today. They've been brainwashed to believe that joy comes from getting something they do *not* have, rather than recognizing and appreciating what they *do* have.

There's probably no better example than the modern Olympic Games to show how this attitude has been carried too far. Competitors who do not win a gold medal, break a world record, or score a perfect 10, seem to be considered unimportant by the public. Their accomplishments are not fully recognized, their success is not fully appreciated, and their names are quickly forgotten. Instant replays and computers show and take apart every move they make, and magnify every mistake. Many dreams are shattered and hearts are broken, not because the achievement wasn't a great one, but because the performance wasn't polished to absolute perfection.

Once the spaceship takes off, the adolescent pioneers will be propelled into an uncertain new frontier, and precarious proving ground. With adults expecting more and more of them, and with friends their own age demanding that they act a certain way, many of the new astronauts will begin to wonder, "Am I made of the right stuff?"

Mother Nature has created a very challenging schedule for adolescents, with certain objectives for growth and development to be finished in a pretty short period of time. In addition to these natural, down-to-earth demands, teenagers must also measure up to modern society's false standards on how to look, feel, and act. This poses a direct threat to their growth as individuals, as well as to their physical and mental wellbeing. Since magazines, television, movies, and other media are constantly telling teenagers that perfection is the most valuable product, it's very easy for young people to get caught up in what may be termed the Perfect 10 syndrome. To look perfect you need to be good looking, have a great body, and wear fashionable clothes. To feel perfect you need to drink booze, smoke dope, or use other chemicals. To act perfect you have to submit to popular opinion, rebel against authority, and join the sexual revolution. Adolescents, in ambitious pursuit of happiness, are very likely to buy into this trap and fall prey to such mistaken thinking. Unfortunately, those who follow this philosophy may be setting themselves up for a life of frustration and failure.

With expectations that are out of this world, it's no wonder that coming of age can grow old real fast. To be true to themselves, teens must learn how to search deep within. It can be hard to sort through the flood of confusing and sometimes false messages that seem to come from everywhere, because the adolescent brain works a little differently than the brain of an adult does.

As teenagers grow up, the way they handle all these outside pressures will be ruled by their own personal values, along with a mixture of what their parents believe, how their friends feel, and the opinions of other important people like relatives, religious leaders, and teachers. All these different beliefs and feelings will blend together to make a very necessary map, or blueprint, for building the inner self.

Building the inner self is a very important goal of adolescence. To reach this goal, there are five main psychological and social jobs that have to be done.

It's easy to remember these five important jobs by thinking of them as the FIVE I's.

1) Creating your own, individual *Identity*.
2) Learning how to act *Independently*.
3) Struggling with your body *Image* (how you feel about how you look).
4) Learning about *Interpersonal* relationships (connections with other people).
5) *Intellectual* awakening (growing from concrete to abstract thinking).

It's important to remember that progress in these five jobs doesn't always happen in order, or smoothly and evenly. Progress also doesn't depend on the person's actual age.

These five accomplishments must also be mixed together with all the fast hormone changes and physical growth that happens, to build the outer self, which is the personality and appearance that the teenager shows to the outside world.

What everybody wants is for teens to stay happy and healthy so they'll have a smooth journey through adolescence, and return safely as tomorrow's adults.

This is our mission!

CHAPTER 2
Fasten Your Seatbelts

Let's begin an imaginary space journey that will describe how teenagers grow up through adolescence. To understand better the mental and social changes that happen, it's helpful to divide adolescence into three main stages.

Think of the launch stage as early adolescence (10 to 14 years old), the orbit stage as middle adolescence (15 to 17 years old), and the reentry stage as late adolescence (18 to 21 years old). These ages are rough estimates, and there can be a lot of overlap. Each teenager is an individual, and will often grow at their own speed, which may be different than others. We all know adolescents who act older or younger than their actual age.

The flight plan for our space journey includes the HEADS FIRST Checklist, as shown on the next page. This checklist is written so it's easy to remember, and it points out today's most important adolescent health care issues. These 10 topics will be talked about in order throughout the book, using the cue words, shown to the right of each topic, to help map out the flight plan.

The HEADS FIRST Checklist*

- **H**ome: Separation, support, space to grow
- **E**ducation: Expectations, study habits, achievement
- **A**buse: Emotional, verbal, physical, sexual
- **D**rugs: Tobacco, alcohol, marijuana, others
- **S**afety: Dangerous activities, seatbelts, helmets

- **F**riends: Confidant, peer pressure, interaction
- **I**mage: Self-esteem, looks, appearance
- **R**ecreation: Exercise, relaxation, TV, media games
- **S**exuality: Changes, feelings, experiences, identity
- **T**hreats: Harm to self or others, running away

*Modified and reproduced with permission of Pediatrics in Review, volume 15, pages 485-489, 1994. *Anticipatory Guidance for the Adolescent: Has It Come of Age?* By Robert M. Cavanaugh Jr., M.D.

The wording of the HEADS FIRST checklist highlights the importance of getting into adolescents' heads as the key to touching their hearts, and helping them cut down on their dangerous, risk-taking behavior. The highlighted letters, shown in the checklist above, will appear at the beginning of each chapter, to guide you through each of the three major growth stages of the space flight: the launch stage, the orbit stage, and the reentry stage.

The 10 topics listed -- home, education, etc. -- are covered in order, one chapter at a time, beginning with the launch stage in Part One of the book. The same pattern is then repeated with the corresponding ten chapters for the orbit stage in Part Two, and the reentry stage in Part Three.

As with any long trip, there is no guarantee of a safe return, and arrival as an adult, right on time, should never be considered automatic. *Dying to be Perfect: How Teens Can Stay Happy, Healthy and Alive* gives a survival plan that will help teenagers and their parents go step-by-step through the basic changes, challenges, and choices that occur during the flight. This book will show both teenagers and parents how to get through the tough times and complete the mission successfully, while still trusting their basic instincts when deciding what the right thing to do is. Real life stories of teenagers (with made-up first names) have been used to make important points. As we are about to see, different adolescents respond very differently in each of the HEADS FIRST categories, as they grow from one stage to the next.

So buckle up, everyone, and get ready to join me on this exciting adventure. It's time to discover what makes the teen tick in search of the Perfect 10.

PART ONE

The Launch
Early Adolescence – 10 to 14 Years

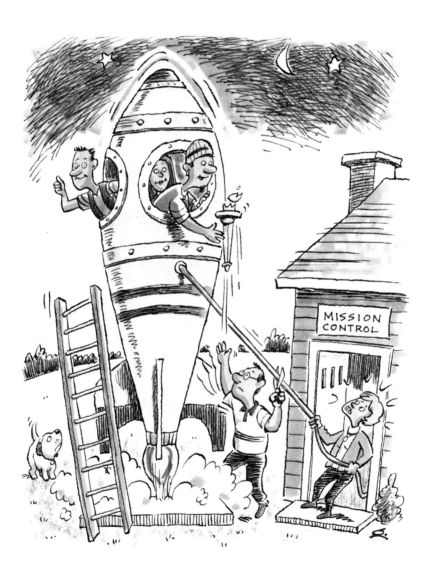

CHAPTER 3
You Have Reached TIME ZERO

Home may be where the heart is, but it's time for adolescents to head out as their separation from home begins. Five, four, three, two, one – they're off. Powered by surging hormones, growth speeds up quickly, generating unique forces and setting off worries about being normal and being accepted. Things do not always happen according to a convenient or well-planned schedule. As the security of childhood is left behind, an emotional emptiness is created at a time when the astronaut still needs guidance and support from his or her parents. To help make this feeling of insecurity and loneliness go away, teenagers want to spend more time with others of their own age and sex. Boys hang out with boys, and girls hang out with girls.

As teens begin to pull at the strings that tie them to their homes, parents who have trouble cutting the cord may be left clinging by a thread. Parents who don't want to let go of their children, or parents who can't let go, may threaten the success of the space flight if they have become too deeply wrapped up in their children's lives.

TEEN TIP - It's tough to raise parents these days. Here are a couple of hints to help you understand where they may be coming from. If you're their first born, you are actually the practice child. They may try out several different parenting methods on you while they try to get it right. One time they may seem too strict, another time too easy. They may not be very consistent, and this may not seem fair. If you're the youngest, then in their eyes it's your job to never grow up. They may struggle with the thought that their baby is about to become a fully-grown adult. Remind them that you are no longer in the cradle, and you don't want to be babied. If you're a middle child, or somewhere in between, you may feel that you're not getting the attention you deserve. If you don't say much, your parents may take for granted that everything is going okay, even if it isn't. This is when you need to speak out, openly and honestly, rather than trying to express your feelings indirectly, through behavior that is not always right.

Even good kids have bad moments. As teens first take off on their flight, they often mistakenly come to believe that they are indestructible. They feel that they will live forever, and that nothing bad can happen to them. Doctors call this belief the 'personal fable.' When teens talk with their friends and find out some of them feel the same way, this just makes their belief stronger.

As peak lift-off velocity is reached, adolescents may suddenly act on impulse, as if they aren't thinking or using good judgement. Their behavior can be unpredictable, almost crazy sometimes, because many can't cool their jets. This is when 'concrete thinking' dominates; adolescents are paying so much attention to what's happening right here and now that they don't seem to be able to think about or understand what might happen to them in the future, because of what they're doing. The expression, "It's now or never," was probably invented by teenagers in the launch stage.

Although this stage usually passes by, some adults still act like they are stuck in it.

This is show time for teens! During the lift-off, adolescents often begin to act as if they're performing on stage in front of an imaginary audience. They believe everyone's eyes are looking at them, wherever they go and whatever they do. Every move they make is meant for this audience.

And during this very sensitive period, teens usually feel that their parents should be neither seen nor heard -- even though their presence must still be felt.

This may cause difficult times for both the teens in flight and the parents back on the ground. Any warning bells that go off from below will probably be mostly ignored by the astronauts. But at the same time it's important that adolescents who are soaring to new heights get a sense that their parents will give them the right help to reach the next level. The reins may need to be pulled a little tighter to help steady those who have too much slack, or loosened up a bit to help calm down those who are getting too uptight. Teens who stay out too late may need to come home earlier, while those who are nervous about going out at all may need to be encouraged, maybe by offering to take them somewhere, or finding activities for them. Some teenagers carry their own safety harness, but others may rely on a safety net, or spotters, for added protection.

As adolescents start to grow up, they may come down with altitude sickness. As they leave the launch pad, they may begin to shake and sway in the crosswinds. Parents may seem puzzled by the wide mood swings that seem to come out of the blue, yet this is all part of the struggle for independence and the search for identity. As parents sit at the control panel, they may wish they could see the whole picture in slow motion, or be able to push the pause button. But very energetic, powerful things are happening. There's usually no time for anyone to bail out, or even take a deep breath. Everything seems to occur with blinding speed, and at a hectic pitch. In the heat of the moment, the ability to stay in tune may seem to scatter like the fumes of a jet's vapor trail.

Sometimes a third party, an outside supporter who is not a member of the family, is needed to help everyone chill out. As a doctor, I keep a 24-hour hotline and have an open-door policy for the families I work with, to help clear the atmosphere of any static or smog. Conference calls and family meetings are particularly useful to settle any differences.

Talking to teens and their parents about family rules, regulations, and restrictions can provide clues about how to untie the knots that are holding the flight down. To live independently, adolescents must be given the right mix of privacy, freedom, and responsibility. "Don't go there" is a good rule for parents to follow, when it comes to understanding that teens need to be able to trade secrets with their friends, and keep their personal space private. Their room should be off limits to any outside intruders, their calls should not be monitored, and controlling their activities should be less and less restrictive as they mature. This is no time for parents to be sniffing around without a good reason. Sometimes teens may need to post a reminder on their door stating, "Invited guests only." The only time a room should be searched, a phone be tapped, or a teenager be followed, is when there is real reason to believe that something harmful might happen, or be happening, to them or to someone else.

Yet as new heights are achieved and rules are made less strict, it must be remembered that young adults still need the support of adults as they search for space to grow.

The process of growing up and becoming mature takes time and effort on everyone's part. There is also an element of 'learn as you go' with such a mission. As their child auditions for adulthood, parents will be taking a test of their own. No one ever said it would be easy to play the role of mother or father. Some parents may want to close their eyes and wake up when it's all over. Others may wish that they could get a sneak preview of what's coming next. Still others may stall for a little extra time, to practice their part. Those who are put on the spot, or who are sitting on the hot seat, can always take a peek at hints or instructions on cue cards left behind by the generations that came before them.

In some ways growing up is like a stage play, with the adult and teenagers playing different parts. When the curtain goes up, parents who feel pressured to perform perfectly may get stage fright. Others may stutter and stammer if the scenes change too fast. And the characters do not always follow the script. Teenagers are famous for making up their own lines, or even doing something completely different than what was in the script. There's no time for retakes or instant replays, so it will be impossible to keep from making some small mistakes. As the plot thickens, it's best to go on with the show and keep the action moving instead of paying too much attention to the mistakes. Very often, these blunders make the best memories, or collections of bloopers, for later reruns. Crazy teenage adventures sometimes become great family stories, told with laughter for a lifetime.

It's tough for parents to stay sharp when they're on duty morning, noon, and night, day in and day out. That would make anyone blurry-eyed. Sleepovers and similar nighttime teenage activities can add to the parents' foggy minds. It's no wonder so many parents put on that extra pot of coffee for a little boost, or even think about popping a few pep pills.

Some situations, though, can be bitter pills to swallow, or make even the best parents hit the boiling point. Marriage problems, work problems, moving to a new house or apartment, or having to take care of their own parents, all add extra stress to parents' lives. Menopause and adolescence are also not a good mix, nor are male mid-life crises and exuberant youthful endeavors.

When these things happen while the teenage astronauts are in their flight, it can push parents over the edge. But they have to stay on call and be available for their teenagers 24 hours a day, 7 days a week, 365 days a year.

PARENT TIP - It's worth it! There is no profession more important than being a mother or a father. This is the opportunity of a lifetime. Being a good parent should always be considered Job One. In this context, the measure of success should be the standard of rearing, not the standard of living.

A useful plan for parents during this stage is to hunker down, but don't hover. They need to be alert, to be aware and to be available, but not overbearing. As mom and dad assume their position at the control panel, they must keep a watchful eye for upcoming events. As they sort through incoming signals, they must be able to recognize when something is about to go wrong. And as they start to pull back from their teenagers, or get pushed away, they must still keep tabs on their kids. In short, parents must still be there as a source of support, even if it's from a distance.

PARENT TIP - The key is to somehow stay connected. Your emotional presence is even more important than your physical presence. It is extremely comforting for teens to know that they can count on you in a crisis, or for simple, everyday problems. For you to fulfill your role as a parent, it takes courage to stand back and let your teen's developmental changes proceed when so many dangers lie ahead. It takes confidence to step aside as the little boy or little girl who once bounced on your knee or blew butterfly kisses begins to spread newly found wings. And, most of all, it takes a commitment to provide roots bound by unconditional love at all times and under all circumstances!

Although these ground rules may not always seem convenient, it's essential for parents to keep communication channels open so they can keep close track of their teen's condition, get a clear reading on any matters which may arise, and respond as needed.

Periodically, there may be blackouts or silent intervals when young crewmembers prefer to trade secrets among themselves. This may leave even the best parents completely in the dark from time to time. In anticipation, many parents will learn to burn the midnight oil so they'll be able to spot any signs of trouble as soon as possible. Other parents may learn to sleep with one eye open so they won't be caught off guard, no matter how late the hour.

Conflict, fighting, or illness at home can cast a shadow over this already-challenging time. However, parents are centrally important in the lives of their children, and it must be completely accepted that teens care about their family. It's not commonly understood or appreciated how much adolescents actually worry about their parents' relationship, as well as the physical and mental health of family members and friends. Teens are very sensitive to such issues, and it must be assumed that they're affected by them. How they deal with this is can be very different from one teen to another, and will depend on each one's individual personality, how mature they are, and how strong their support systems are. Depending on the circumstances, their responses may range from coming right out and saying something about their concerns, to letting parents know that they're worried by coming down with physical problems that don't seem to have clear causes.

Although adolescents are masters of communication, they're also well known for their hidden agenda. Their messages may be written between the lines, and interpreting their body language may be an art in itself. Deciphering the code may sometimes seem as mysterious as reading tea leaves. It's important to involve all significant family members, to provide meaningful insight in situations where teens seem to be struggling and having difficulty getting their point across to others. In certain situations, an experienced health professional may be needed to help sort out the signs and symptoms in an effort to help parents, as well as their kids, grow up. The following cases will illustrate this point.

Caught in a crossfire

Janet was a 12-year-old girl trapped in the middle of a bitter custody battle between her mother and father. She was also the middle child, with an older and a younger sister. The parents had separated, but still lived near one another so that the girls could shuffle back and forth between them rather easily. Janet was referred to me by a pediatrician who was treating her for an eating disorder. Janet was under enormous stress, and losing a lot of weight. Her condition was so serious it was threatening her life, and she required medical stabilization.

I performed a thorough investigation, and agreed with the diagnosis of anorexia. It was obvious to our staff that Janet was the one who had taken on the job of keeping peace in the family, and was desperately trying to hold everyone together. The worse the fighting became, and the more the family seemed to fall apart, the less Janet ate.

Mom and dad were told that their daughter's illness put her life at risk, and they stopped attacking each other and started treating each other more politely. After three weeks of intensive inpatient psychiatric treatment, Janet had gained back enough weight so that she was no longer in immediate danger. That's when the hard work really started.

I enlisted the support of a child and adolescent psychiatrist. We followed the family for several months in an outpatient family therapy setting. Things really got ugly at times, with frequent, heated arguments between the mother and father. We could only imagine the stress and turmoil that the girls faced at home. The parents were never really able to bury the hatchet. They were both very good people, but they just could not get along. They were constantly running each other down in front of us, and it was easy to get a picture of what was going on at home. The mother was particularly resentful of the father's extramarital exploits, and she made no bones about this in front of the kids. She was especially offended, and probably a little jealous, about him bringing his companions to his house when the girls were around. Dad would then launch a counterattack of his own. This would go on an on, session after session. Janet had to deal with this every day.

We offered suggestions to help Janet deal with this, and she was able to keep busy with many activities, including ballet. She realized that ballet placed her at further risk with her eating disorder, because of the extreme importance put on being thin in this sport. But ballet was an important outlet for her, and with encouragement from our nutritionist she was gradually able to balance her food intake and energy expenditure in a healthier way. She began to realize that she had her own life to lead, and that it was not her fault that her parents could not get along. It was also not her job to solve the problems and disagreements between them. It took a long three years, but Janet was able to make a complete recovery. During this difficult time, the parents were able to stay connected with their daughters and to show their love for them. The girls, in turn, obviously felt the same way about their parents. Without everyone staying connected and showing their love, this story may not have had such a good outcome.

Calling for a cease fire

Tina was a 13-year-old girl who developed a stomach pain in connection with a mild flu-like illness. The pain was rather vague, and located throughout her abdomen. Although the flu infection was completely gone in a few days, the pain stayed. She was given a complete medical examination, and everything seemed physically normal. But her pain still did not go away, so I continued to keep an eye on her.

Tina finally told me that she was very worried about the relationship between her parents, who were going to separate. Tina's parents were very concerned about their daughter's health, and it was noticed that both parents pulled together to help her while she was sick. It was realized that Tina's stomach pain made the parents put off splitting up. They were able to temporarily forget their disagreements and gather around Tina when she was in sick bay. So there was a good mental reason for Tina to hold on to a physical problem. As long as her stomach hurt, her parents did not separate.

It's not unusual for teenagers to behave this way and develop physical problems when there is trouble between the parents. But it's important to point out that these teens don't always do it on purpose, and usually don't even realize why they're doing it.

Once Tina went into therapy and learned new ways of dealing with her parents' plans to split up, her pain gradually went away. At last contact, her parents were still together, but it appeared that they were about to head their separate ways.

More than shouldering the burden

This was a similar case of abdominal pain in a 13-year-old girl whose parents were splitting up. Maggie developed sharp, knife-like cramps in the right upper portion of her abdomen, and the cramps reached all the way up into the right shoulder. The pain would begin suddenly, and it stayed in the same place. The surgeon consulted with me because his studies, even those of the gallbladder, were all normal, and he was concerned that there might be a mental reason for the pain, caused by the family situation.

After I did a very thorough evaluation it was obvious to me that Maggie was adjusting as well as could be expected to her parents' marriage problems. In fact, she actually felt some relief that they were splitting up, because things had been too tense at home. I could not find any other obvious source of stress.

Important clues to the problem's answer were the facts that the pain always occurred in the same place, it came on suddenly, and it was sharp and stabbing. These features are not typically seen in patients with mental reasons for having abdominal pain. All the signs still pointed to the gallbladder.

A doctor who specialized in the stomach and intestines did a special study and found out that Maggie's gallbladder was not normal. It was removed, and Maggie's pain disappeared.

This case points out that it should never be assumed that stomach pain or other such symptoms have a purely mental cause, just because teens are under stress or living in a confused situation.

The mom who had one too many

Danielle was a 13-year-old girl referred to me by her family doctor. She had pain in her large joints, including the elbows, hips, knees and ankles. There was no swelling, redness, limitation of motion, or other signs of arthritis. I ordered some more tests, in addition to the ones her family doctor had done, but all the results came back negative. There was no sign of any physical problem.

When Danielle came back for a follow-up visit I asked her to fill out the personal questionnaire that I routinely use. Her answers to the questions were very striking and emotional. She came right out and said that her home was in total confusion, with arguments and yelling all the time. Her mother was an alcoholic, and the woman was upsetting the entire household. Danielle bore the brunt of her mother's anger, and the girl no longer knew what to do about it. She had nobody to talk to about it, and had thought about running away to escape from the complete confusion.

Unlike Maggie, whose pain had a physical cause, it was obvious that Danielle had nothing wrong physically. It seemed to me that severe, ongoing stress was the most likely reason for her joint pain, so I referred her to a therapist. The girl was very grateful that she had someone to talk openly to, and for the first time tell about her frustrations. Alcohol treatment for the mother, and counseling for the other family members, was also recommended.

This case shows how problems at home can be a leading source of stress and anxiety among adolescents. Teenagers often worry about their parents' relationship, as well as the physical and mental health of other family members. It's important to point out that more than 20 percent of boys and girls in a recent study at our center believed that a family member had a problem with alcohol or other drugs. Very often, though, it is hard for adolescents to come right out and talk about these worries directly. Such feelings are often kept inside and told to no one. Then they may be expressed indirectly, by coming down with vague physical symptoms.

Pain is only one of many ways this happens. Although headaches and stomach discomfort are pretty common, it is not unusual to have pain in the extremities, such as the arms or legs, as in Danielle's case. Adolescents who have no one to talk to about conflict, fighting, abusive behavior, or similar problems at home are at very high risk for running away or expressing their distress through other potentially dangerous acting-out behaviors. Repressed memories that do not show up until adulthood may also occur.

Friends and loved ones who wish to help reduce the emotional burden of youth must be willing to listen without judgement, and to encourage open discussions on these family issues. Sometimes these listeners may need to get beyond their own denial about what's happening in the family, before they can help adolescents deal with their personal struggles.

Cupid and the convict

Tammy was a 14-year-old girl who had experienced vague stomach pain for several months. Her physical exam was completely normal and all studies came up with nothing. It was obvious that something was bothering Tammy, and as I got to know her a little better, she was able to tell me that she was under a lot of stress. It turned out that her father was about to be released from prison. He had been threatening Tammy and her mother so much that they feared for their lives. They had gone to great lengths to make their home secure, and the mother's new boyfriend had even bought a gun to help defend them. This made everyone tense and anxious. Tammy was so stressed out that she was developing real physical symptoms because of her emotional turmoil. It was very obvious that she and her mother were having a hard time dealing with the situation.

The story then took a very interesting turn when the father made several friendly phone calls to Tammy and her mother after he got out of jail. He soon began seeing them again on a more regular basis, and fortunately their worst fears never came true. Instead, the parents' relationship became so good that they actually got back together, and the boyfriend moved out. Since the father had been shot with Cupid's bow and arrow, there was no longer any need for the gun.

At my last contact with the family everything was fine, and Tammy seemed happy and pain-free.

★★★★★★

Life is no fun for the child who has to take on the chores of being an adult at too early an age. It's hard to find the right mix of freedom and responsibility. In addition to the normal work of growing up, going to school, and doing the usual household chores, these teens have to take on the added duty of acting like a parent too. They may have to take care of younger brothers or sisters, or family members who are sick, disabled, or handicapped, while one or both parents work to put enough food on the table. This is especially true when a single parent needs to have extra jobs just to make enough money to survive, and a teen has to take up the slack at home. Many of these adolescents are also forced to get jobs of their own to bring in extra money for the family. Few if any, will have any spending money left over for themselves.

Young adolescents respond in different ways to being forced to grow up too soon. Some accept it, some don't. They all still need to be a kid. Whenever possible, these teens should be allowed to have a little time for themselves. Most are very grateful for such consideration, and do not take advantage of it.

In contrast, those who are not given enough freedom may react very negatively. This must be recognized so that adolescents who have more limits are able to get their frustrations out before they act out in socially unacceptable ways. I have seen many teens who engaged in sexual activity, abused drugs, or took other risks because they had a hard time dealing with daily routines loaded with work. Some even activated the ejection button to escape the pressure, and ran away from home.

It is especially important for families that already have too much to do, to understand that giving everyone a little break can offer a big payback, even when it is fit into very demanding schedules. It is possible for the mission to be completed successfully if they are all able to pull together and work as a team. Such an achievement will be worth more than the time it takes away from the schedule, and it will make everyone in the family feel like they've accomplished something.

CHAPTER 4
School Daze

Education and academics put teens to the test. However, there is much more to mental growth than simply getting book knowledge or good grades. Widening of the thought processes, learning how to look into the future, and developing a sensitivity toward other people, are all in the lesson plan. As the launch proceeds, there is a new sense of purpose for enthusiastic young people who set out to save the world with their idealistic goals and ambitions. Maybe they are slightly ahead of their time, or maybe society should pay attention, because teens usually have good ideas that come from their hearts.

In their search for peace and harmony, there is always concern that over-excited teens will overshoot the target, while others may not have the energy needed to finish the job. Schools may be seen as a steadying influence during these times, and are often used as temporary guardians. But not everyone does well in an academic or structured environment. In many cases the neutral ground of the classroom is not as smooth as it is supposed to be. While some students may be able to fit in fine and toe the mark, others may stumble on the unforgiving surface. Still others may play hooky, cut classes, or show up late whenever possible. For many teens, school-related issues become a leading source of stress and anxiety. These feelings may not be obvious at first, and they may not seem to be related to school. In fact they may not even be visible. But over time, the effects of this stress and anxiety can build up and take a heavy toll on teens.

Because of this, it's important that teens be screened for problems at school on a regular basis. Hooking up with a medical module for regular checkups is an excellent way to take a close, fair look at how things are going. As part of such a routine exam, I ask teens if they like school, if they ever had to repeat a grade, or if they are currently having any trouble with their classes. Absences because of illness are another important thing to take a close look at.

It also helps to find out if teens think that their performance meets with everyone's hopes, and that everyone approves of it. Very often, their achievements may not be as good as they, their parents, or their teachers had expected it to be. This may cause a lot of anxiety and tension, especially in teens who expect a lot of themselves, or who are expected to do too much. Sometimes adults have unreasonably high hopes for their children. It's important to find out which teens are working on overload before things get too hot, sparks begin to fly, or someone gets burned. For this reason I carry an ample supply of fuses, circuit breakers and safety switches on hand in the office. In most cases, it's simply a matter of talking things through with the family and getting everyone back on track with a quick reality check. Occasionally, more intense short-term medical intervention is needed to stop a crisis.

TEEN TIP - Sometimes it may seem as if you just can't do anything right. Although you may fail at certain things, this does not mean that you are a failure as a person. It simply means that you are not perfect. While this may come as a bit of a shock to you, take comfort in the fact that nobody else is, either. Whenever you suffer any setbacks, take a little break to regroup, re-examine what you want to accomplish, and set your sights on tomorrow. Learning how to pick yourself up after you fall down is what growing up is all about.

The vanishing fatigue syndrome

Sonya was a 13-year-old girl referred to me because she had had a flu-like illness a month ago, and even though the infection was gone, she was still tired all the time. A complete medical examination showed that there was nothing physically wrong with her.

She had not been able to go to school since the illness began. This caused trouble at home because her father thought she was healthy enough to go to school, but her mother thought she should be allowed to stay at home until she felt better. The problem was made worse by the fact that both parents were teachers, and they were from different schools of thought on child rearing.

Sonya looked healthy, but for some reason she did not want to go to school. I was able to talk her into sitting in her parents' car in the school parking lot, as long as she didn't have to go inside. She was able to do this without any problem. Next I was able to persuade her to sit in the school nurse's office for two hours a day. She was also able to do this without any trouble. But she still didn't want to go into a regular classroom.

I told the mother that since Sonya was physically able to go to school in a limited way, I felt she was tired because she had a deep fear of school itself. But the mother would not even consider the possibility that her daughter was developing a school phobia.

After doing some research on the Internet, the mother believed that Sonya had chronic fatigue syndrome. I told the parents that Sonya did not meet the requirements to have this problem. People with chronic fatigue syndrome are tired for at least six months, and Sonya had been this way only one month.

The family decided to see another doctor, who was an expert on chronic fatigue. After a quick visit, Sonya was told she did have chronic fatigue syndrome. The doctor said this even though there were no guidelines for this condition in adolescents at the time, and Sonya had been sick for less than the six months, the minimum time required to decide whether adults had this condition.

Much to her delight, Sonya was tutored at home for the last few weeks of the school year. This lowered her anxiety about school a lot, because she no longer felt overwhelmed. She was able to work at her own speed with the tutor, and finally caught up with all her schoolwork, and passed all her classes.

Usually, it's best to cure a fear of school by having the student go back to school as soon as possible. Occasionally, as in Sonya's case, teenagers get so far behind that personal, one-on-one help from a tutor is needed to help them catch up and get their confidence back.

Later that summer Sonya's mother called me and asked if I could call in a prescription for her daughter's sunburn. When I asked how Sonya got the sunburn, her mom said that she had been playing outside all day long for two weeks, in a roller hockey league. We both laughed, because it was obvious that Sonya had made a pretty dramatic recovery. The last time I talked to her family, her energy level was back to normal and she was able to return to school that fall on a full time basis.

Getting off to a fresh start seemed to be the only cure that was needed. So much for the diagnosis of chronic fatigue syndrome in this case!

The hacker and his honey

Vinny was an 11-year-old boy who was referred to me because of a dry, hacking cough that wouldn't go away. He had been a healthy boy until he developed repeated breathing problems associated with asthma over the past year. An in-depth medical exam found no physical reason for his symptoms. He had been on many medications, but the coughing wouldn't stop. This was a real problem at night because it kept Vinny and everyone else in the house awake. The cough also kept him from doing much during the day, and it even bothered other students during class at school. His chest also hurt, and he was tired all the time. He had missed three months of school because of these symptoms.

Vinny's doctor and guidance counselors were convinced that his cough was somehow connected to the fact that he seemed very nervous about being in school. Doctors call this a "psychogenic" cough. It is important to understand that this type of cough is usually not done on purpose, and most adolescents are not able to deliberately control it. The key is to decide whether the cough actually is psychogenic. If it is, it can be treated by getting rid of, or lessening, the anxiety that is causing it.

We did a physical examination in our office, and Vinny seemed to be a fairly healthy boy. He had some difficulty breathing through his nose, and some mild tenderness over his chest. The rest of his exam was completely normal. I also talked with Vinny alone, and I could not discover any stress factors or reasons for him not wanting to go to school. In fact, he missed his teachers and his girlfriend at school. He seemed to be very well adjusted, and even a bit laid back. What little anxiety he did show appeared to be a result of the cough, rather than the cause of it. Something seemed to be missing here, and it soon became obvious that we needed to do a little more detective work.

The pediatric resident assigned to Vinny's case and I then reviewed the previous X-ray films with our radiologist. It was then apparent that Vinny had signs of significant sinusitis, which had somehow been missed. The postnasal drip associated with this condition could explain the cough, which was especially uncomfortable at night. A psychogenic cough, however, is not likely to occur when the patient is sleeping. The radiologist had accurately described the problem, but another specialist who was involved in Vinny's case had misunderstood the radiologist's original report. The specialist then passed this misinformation to Vinny's pediatrician, who was never aware of the need to treat Vinny with antibiotics.

The resident looked at me and said, "You don't suppose the sinus infection could be causing the persistent cough, do you?"

I then called the pediatrician, and we put Vinny on antibiotics. He came back two weeks later and was completely cured. The chest pain from the repetitive coughing had also disappeared. His mother was thrilled, and Vinny was delighted to be back in school. His only complaint was that his girlfriend was now sick, and he was very upset that he was still unable to see her.

We may have cured Vinny of his sinus infection, but we don't have any way to treat people bitten by the love bug.

★★★★★★

Physical handicaps and illnesses that last a long time can be a real challenge to young people who are maturing. They can also make academic achievement difficult. Unusual stresses that are building up in a teen's unconscious mind can blow up and endanger the process of maturing. There must be a way for that teen to blow off steam about any hidden worries they have. There should also be extra support for them, to make their lives more stable during their journey to adulthood.

But it is not appropriate, and it does not help, to treat handicapped or sick teens as if they are weak, frail, or fragile. They are not looking for anyone's pity or sympathy. They also do not want, or deserve, to be treated as different from others their age. It must be recognized that while they may have special medical needs, they also face the same day-to-day pressures as their healthier peers.

PARENT TIP – Be protective, but not overprotective. The goal is to teach affected teens how to rely on themselves for their sense of worth, rather than others. They should not be sheltered from information on important adolescent health issues such as substance abuse, sexuality, self-esteem, safety and stress. Open discussions on these topics at home, at school, or in the doctor's office are more than just preventative for teenagers with chronic medical conditions. They also provide this group with a feeling of being included, which helps them keep their sense of dignity as individuals.

CHAPTER 5
Staying Out of Harm's Way

Abuse is one of the most sensitive issues for adolescents to discuss. The importance of extending a helping hand to those who may have been victimized cannot be underestimated. More than 700,000 women are raped each year, and approximately 60% of them are 19 years of age or younger. In addition, although teenagers account for nearly 50% of reported cases of abused children, it is difficult for them to complain or tell anyone about it by themselves, without someone asking them about it. This is particularly true for the large number of adolescents whose only medical exam is a sports physical, which is often done when they are with many other people, in an assembly line atmosphere. It is best to ask for sensitive or classified information in more protected, private surroundings. There may be no actual physical proof of any reported abuse, but the teenager's own feelings about what happened during such traumatic experiences must be identified and dealt with as soon as possible, to prevent the distress or injury from continuing. Waiting for SOS signals, or until suspicions have become very high, which is how it used to be done, can put off recognizing the abuse, and doing something to stop it. Thus, it has been recommended by leading authorities in the field that routine screening and monitoring for abuse be built into the adolescent's medical file.

PARENT TIP - Don't be an enabler. Turning your head the other way and ignoring abuse only serves to help it continue. Any apparent benefits in the short run will usually carry a big long-term cost. Protecting a spouse or other family member from outside scrutiny should never be given a higher priority than your teen's health and happiness.

As a doctor, I feel that I have to talk with teens about abuse and other sensitive health-related topics. To accomplish this I ask them to fill out a personal questionnaire. They do this privately in my office. I then go over the form confidentially with them.

In the questionnaire, the issue of abuse is simply asked about as follows: "Has anyone ever abused you by their actions or their words? If yes, please check all forms of abuse that apply: physical ... sexual ... emotional ... verbal ... other ... " In a recent survey in our center, more than 40% of both boys and girls said that they had been abused or mistreated in some way. It is also remarkable that 18% of the girls who filled out the questionnaire revealed that they had been sexually abused. It is striking that none of these girls were being seen for suspected abuse. They also had said nothing to anybody about the abuse, until they were asked in the questionnaire.

The fact that so many girls said they were sexually abused means this issue must be looked at more closely. The short-term results and long-term complications for victims of such acts are known to be very severe. The perpetrator of the abuse is frequently a close family member, or other person well known to the adolescent. It should not be too surprising that teenagers feel that dealing with sexual abuse is very important in health care. This topic also ranks very high on the parents' agenda for routine adolescent health care. The same is true of physical, emotional, and verbal abuse.

In many instances, however, teenagers are too shy, embarrassed, or even afraid to disclose such issues on their own and hope that others will discover their plight. Adolescents and their families often give the job of discovering the problem, and doing something about it, to medical professionals.

Sinking into a slump

Ricky was a 12-year-old boy who came to our office for a routine physical exam. He had recently moved from California to live with his mother, after his parents had separated. Ricky was a shy kid who hung his head low and looked at the floor while he talked. He seemed very timid and insecure. His physical exam was entirely normal, besides the fact that he had mild *scoliosis* (a curve in the spine).

But when he completed the personal questionnaire he related that his father had constantly insulted him and treated him with contempt, often for no obvious reason. It soon became evident that Ricky's self-esteem had been beaten down, and that he was suffering from deep emotional wounds. In fact, he even blamed himself for having scoliosis. His father had frequently insulted him for not standing perfectly straight, and had warned Ricky that if he slouched, his spine would be deformed.

As is usually the case, the cause of Ricky's scoliosis was found to be completely unknown. We explained to him that his mild back deformity was not caused by anything he did or did not do. It was hard for us to convince him, because he had been trained to think badly of himself, and blame himself for any problem. This is very typical of children and adolescents who have been abused continuously for a long time; they have been made to feel that they are the ones to blame whenever something goes wrong.

Ricky's case illustrates that although verbal and emotional abuse may not always be reportable, it can have a serious impact on young, unprotected targets. In fact, it can be just as painful as physical and sexual abuse and in some instances be even more traumatizing to teenagers. Treatment is directed at rebuilding self-esteem and promoting self-confidence over a period of time. There is no substitute for continued love and support to satisfy such needs. Ricky's mother clearly understood this, and he started to do really well as she supported, complimented, and nurtured him.

★★★★★★

Sometimes adolescents may even believe that it's best to keep things secret and let them stay the way they are. They may be afraid that if the authorities find out, they may do things that will be worse than what is already happening. This is particularly true of teens that are just starting out and learning about the outside world. They often fear the unknown, and may be willing to pay the price for whatever security they now have. Many have heard stories of brothers and sisters being separated, and of families split up by the system. Other stories tell of teens being placed in "safe" homes or institutions that turn out to be even worse than the homes the teens came from. These young people may choose the path of least resistance and suffer in silence.

TEEN TIP – If you have been abused, coming forward to tell someone may be one of the most difficult decisions you will ever have to make. Try to understand that the goal is to keep you safe and to keep your family together, whenever possible.

While it is far from perfect, the system for rescuing teens who are in over their head is also by no means useless. Concerned individuals or those who are supposed to report any problems may feel they have to blow the whistle. Sometimes a safety drill alone will be enough, while occasionally a complete removal is necessary. Custody battles are never pretty, nor are battered children. Setting false alarms can be just as ugly and create just as much harm as the supposed abuse. Special forces may need to be called in to help sort out the details. A squad of protective service workers is always on call and ready to respond on a moment's notice. Most are truly dedicated public servants who have grown used to keeping long hours in the field, by day and by night. They get little recognition and even lower wages. They must be saluted, supported, and somehow be able to increase their ranks, because they are in very short supply!

When the watchdog bites its master

Gus was a 10-year-old boy whose parents had recently divorced. He and his 8-year-old brother lived nearby with their mother, and spent every other weekend with their father. This arrangement worked out fairly well until the mother moved 200 miles away. The boys continued to visit the father on the assigned weekends, although this was more difficult due to the long distance now separating them.

The father would often get up at 4 o'clock in the morning so that he could be at his sons' Saturday morning baseball games in the summer and soccer games in the fall.

Shortly before the next Thanksgiving holiday, the father was told by a social worker that the boys would not be visiting him any more, because the mother reported that he had physically abused them.

No doctor had done an examination to prove or disprove the mother's accusation. The father was devastated and did not know what to do or where to turn. He was not allowed to see his boys that Thanksgiving and was only allowed a limited 2-hour supervised visit in cold, sterile surroundings for the Christmas holiday that year. He also had to make many trips out of town to meet with lawyers, psychologists, and social workers, all at his own expense.

After months of struggling and fighting with the legal system it was determined that the accusations against the father were not true, and that there was no basis to the claims made by the mother. The father was then gradually allowed to visit his sons regularly. It turned out that he and his sons had been victims of a plot dreamed up by his ex-wife. They were also victims of a society that was poorly equipped to deal with a real family crisis in a reasonable amount of time. The right resources must be ready for rapid response teams to go to work immediately in such situations. Any accusations must be checked out right away in an effort to avoid any unnecessary pain and suffering for all parties involved. The safety, protection and well being of innocent children and adolescents must always be the top priority.

As part of this plan, special attention should be paid in custody battles over children, because the hateful filing of phony reports of abuse seems to be skyrocketing. This seems to be done so one spouse can get the upper hand over another. Using kids as pawns in such situations must be discouraged rather than encouraged, like it is now, by an old-fashioned legal system that is no longer correct for today's modern times. Parents who make up stories of abuse for their own personal gain must be made to pay for their actions, and no longer be allowed to get away with it. People who make false claims of abuse would probably not be so quick to cause such pain, if they were to feel the same type of shame because of the close look that the law would take at them and their actions. This would be especially true if there was a chance they would get the same punishment for lying, as are those whom they accuse wrongfully.

Although most children's protective workers are dedicated, most judges are not known for their compassion or caring. They can be sheltered in isolated chambers, and putter along, seemingly oblivious to a family's desperate cries for help. Busy schedules with outrageous delays seem to make money for lawyers and other third parties, while using up the energy and money of the people they are supposed to be helping. Such a legal process is a form of abuse and neglect all by itself.

This is a case of the watchdog biting its master. Those who cause this unnecessary pain and suffering must be held accountable to the public that they serve. If they are unable to behave in a more civilized manner they should be put on a shorter leash, reported to the dogcatcher, or even sent to the pound! In other words, the people who voted these judges in should demand better guidelines from Congress and expect the judges to enforce them. Or vote them out of office if they don't.

CHAPTER 6

Getting into the Spirits

D rugs do not mix well with the teenagers' natural desire to experiment. With proper insulation, the spaceship cabin should serve as an isolation chamber to help shield young adolescents from any outside vices or temptations. However, life within the protective walls of the shuttle can still be a mixed bag. Contraband may be easily stashed, stowed or smuggled on board. Sometimes free samples are left around the quarters by previous generations. Curious teens can easily sneak a smoke, take a swig, or even get liquored up under such conditions. Those who seek greater excitement may start to scrounge around in search of higher adventure. They may also be tricked into sponging off an older sponsor who seems to be generous, but who is actually providing the drugs and booze with many strings attached.

TEEN TIP - Nicotine and alcohol are considered gateway drugs. If you enjoy smoking and drinking you have already taken the bait. The farther you go the tougher it gets to turn it around and stay out of the trap. The sooner you come to grips with this the better. The next step is abuse of illegal street drugs, or even a life of addiction.

Sometimes the astronauts may try to crack open the window, hoping to sniff any fumes given off by the giant rocket boosters. Abuse of volatile inhalants such as glue, gasoline, lighter fluid, room odorizers, paint thinner, or other solvents reaches a peak in 8th graders. These substances are especially attractive to young adolescents because they are inexpensive, easy to get, and give a quick high. Unfortunately, most teens do not realize the serious damage these chemicals can do to their body.

The first effect is liveliness and excitation. If the inhaling continues, the central nervous system becomes weighed down. As the poisons begin to build up in the body, seizures, coma, and sudden 'sniffing death' can occur at any point. This can happen even when these substances are breathed in for the first time. Repeated inhaling can also cause serious harm to the brain, heart, lungs, liver, kidneys, and other vital organs.

PARENT TIP – Parents need to be aware that inhalant abuse is relatively common in the 10- to 14-year-old age group. These substances are usually 'sniffed' directly from the container, 'huffed' from a rag or handkerchief soaked in the substance, or placed in a bag and the fumes repeatedly inhaled. Parents should be alert to the possibility of inhalant abuse if they find any leftover bags, pieces of cloth, or other such materials lying around. The unexpected appearance or disappearance of cans, tubes, or other containers of volatile substances should also cause suspicion.

Some may wonder if this generation is going to pot. As with the generation of teenagers that grew up before them, getting high on marijuana continues to be a popular pastime among young explorers. They do this to feel good, to feel perfect, and to make life happy all the time. Getting stoned is not hard to do. Weed is readily available and can be bought by the bag at a cheap price in today's market. Care packages may also be sent up to the space ship by drug dealers just dying to sell their products to unsuspecting prey. These predators know that most such gifts are eagerly opened. Very few are marked return to sender and shipped back. Free pipes and other drug paraphernalia may also be included, at no extra charge.

It must be pointed out that no grade of pot should be considered safe. There is always the risk of contamination. Any of the goods can have impurities mixed in, which can send the user on a bad trip. Getting high is also one of the first steps to getting hooked. It's never too soon to help teens who are using marijuana to put out the fire and see the light before they are sentenced to life on the dark side.

Cheap, convenient, over-the-counter medications such as diet pills or decongestants are completely legal and often used to get a quick buzz. They may also cause a quick blowout, by raising the blood pressure high enough to cause a stroke. Prescription drugs are another handy source of entertainment, and are often passed out at parties for fun. Some teens pass them around to make themselves popular. Cocaine, heroin and similar illegal drugs may hit the scene by early puberty. Tripping out is still in, because LSD and similar drugs are still very available to teenagers. Psychedelic mushrooms, or 'shrooms,' are also commonly abused because they give a hallucinogenic effect. In general, use of such street drugs becomes a more serious problem among older teens, although young adolescents may accidentally wander into a drop-off zone and quickly get in over their heads.

The headache that blew her mind

Kathy was a 14-year-old girl who had been diabetic for several years. She was a very energetic, enthusiastic girl who was also very independent, which sometimes frustrated her doctors. She generally ate whatever she felt like, and often would not take her insulin when she was supposed to. It is not surprising that she often got into trouble with high blood sugar, which required emergency medical treatment. Kathy was also a bit of an experimenter, and began using diet pills, which she had bought in a drugstore. She would take several tablets at a time, trying to get high.

I was called in to see her when she developed a severe, pounding headache. She thought it was another bad migraine because it felt like the migraines she had had before. This time, though, Kathy also had a slight slurring of her speech. Her blood pressure was very high too. Fortunately, treatment quickly brought it down. We then did a CAT scan of her brain and found out that she had had a mild stroke. It was decided that the stroke was caused by the abnormally high blood pressure, which was in turn caused by her abuse of the diet pills.

Kathy recovered completely, but she was very lucky that her stroke had not been a real disaster, damaging her for life. She was also very frightened by the stroke and stopped using drugs, because she did not want to become paralyzed or otherwise crippled.

In spite of the fact that she was very stubborn, Kathy gradually grew to realize that she could control her diabetes, although she could not cure it. Years later I ran into her again one day. A strange thing had happened - she had grown up. She thanked me for helping her, and said that she had been taking good care of herself. It was obvious that her life had taken a turn for the better, and it was very rewarding to have shared in this process.

The girl who was up and down

Dana was a 14-year-old girl referred to me by a family doctor because she kept fainting. The doctor thought Dana should try tilt-table testing, a method that was popular at the time for finding out if the patient had unusually low blood pressure, which might be causing the fainting.

As part of a complete medical history, Dana filled out our personal questionnaire. On it she mentioned that she had used antidepressant medication several times, to get high. In fact, these pills were being passed out at several parties she had recently gone to. When she got home from the party she would take a shower, get light-headed, and pass out.

It was soon obvious that every time she had fainted it was directly related to abuse of the antidepressant medication. No further medical testing was necessary. Dana had not made the connection between the drugs and her fainting, probably because there was usually a several hour delay from the time she took the pills until she had this unpleasant side effect. The fainting frightened her, and her symptoms completely disappeared as soon as she stopped abusing the medication. For Dana, this was a real wake-up call. Her story illustrates how prescription drugs are being abused by adolescents, and how their side effects may sometimes sneak into the picture.

CHAPTER 7
Personal Chauffeurs and Body-guards Needed

S afety for young astronauts should not be left to chance. While it may seem like parents are only needed as a transportation service, or as chaperones, they must grab the opportunity to drive safety messages home to their teens. This is a good time for those in mission control to review basic principles of highway safety. This includes wearing seatbelts, avoiding hitchhiking, and the hazards of alcohol.

Knowledge alone is not enough to get these points across; the equipment and support to do so are also necessary. For example, there should be working seatbelts in the parents' vehicle, and the engine should not be started until all passengers are buckled up. Teens should always be discouraged from thumbing for a ride, and should not be left in a position where they may feel forced to do so.

PARENT TIP – The influence of parents as the most important role models must never be underestimated, especially during this sensitive period when young adolescents still need extra guidance and protection. Even when everything seems to be going in one ear and out the other, it is often surprising to see how much common sense actually sinks in. Patience and persistence do pay off, and they are usually greatly appreciated further down the line.

Unfortunately, teens may become trapped by their own denial, since they truly believe that nothing can happen to them. It doesn't take much to get them going in the thrill-seeking department. All they need to do is just give one another the high sign, and they're off to the races. With so many temptations during the spaceship launch it's easy to get in over their heads before they realize they've gone above and beyond their limits. They often take their miniaturized personal spacecraft (their own or their parents' off-road vehicles) for adventures into virgin territory. This has created a significant impact on our national injury and death statistics, because many young adolescents do not have the necessary physical or maturational skills to operate these vehicles safely. Even before the orbital plateau is reached they often sneak off on their own, doing wheelies with little or no instruction or supervision. Poor laws and a general lack of safety courses only add to this problem. The all-terrain vehicle has recently joined the group of land rovers, and has quickly become a leading cause of injuries to adolescents who may wander off to parts unknown. The jet ski has also plunged right into the market, and made a splash with a wave of accidents over the nation's lakes, rivers, and other bodies of water. That old standby, the snowmobile, still adds more than its share of accidents on ice and snow, too. Although the right laws for these vehicles may not yet be in sight, there is no shortcut when it comes to knowing the common sense rules of the road, the land, or the sea.

Wearing protective headgear while driving any of these off-road vehicles, as well as when riding on a bike or motorcycle, is a basic idea that must be understood, and accepted, by all adolescents. However, it may seem unnatural or meaningless to many of them at this stage. A crash course that teaches a thorough and specific understanding of the operation and safety features of these vehicles is essential before using them. The importance of not driving such craft while drinking or drugging must also be stressed.

TEEN TIP - While it may seem like you cannot be hurt at this age, you don't need to be a hardhead about it. Always wear a helmet to soften the blow in case of an accident. This simple politeness will spare the object you hit from any unnecessary cracks, dents, or other damage. Oh, by the way, your brain will also be given some extra protection at the same time.

The different types of exercise, sports, or forms of recreation will need their own safety precautions. For example, learning how to swim is a fundamental principle of water safety. Swimming with a partner (even in areas with a lifeguard) is another standard safeguard. So is swimming without drinking or using other drugs. Coast Guard-approved life vests and other appropriate floatation devices should always be used for water sports such as canoeing, motor boating, and jet skiing. The rapid increase in adolescent injuries from bouncing on backyard trampolines raises serious questions about private recreational use of this type of device. In addition, helmets are recommended for activities like skateboarding, in-line skating, and riding on scooters.

PARENT TIP – Parents should be aware of the fact that the frequent occurrence of even minor injuries, although not life-threatening, should always arouse suspicion of substance abuse.

As we have been made painfully aware, school safety has become a major issue in recent years. Aside from major acts of violence, which make the headlines, there are everyday problems that can cause a lot of anxiety among younger adolescents. Usually teenagers are able to settle smaller conflicts or disagreements on their own. Sometimes, though, they may need to vent their frustration, fear, or anger to others, to get relief. Sometimes continuing problems may show themselves with unexplained physical symptoms that do not appear to have an emotional basis. The following case is an example.

The bully on the bus

Brad was a 12-year-old boy referred to us because he had recently lost the ability to walk. His pediatrician had done a thorough physical exam and could not come up with an explanation. Brad was then transferred to our hospital for further evaluation and treatment.

He was seen by a number of doctors, and several more investigative studies were done. No actual evidence of any physical abnormality could be found, and once again no one could come up with an explanation. This only seemed to add to everyone's anxiety. Of course his parents were rightfully concerned that their son had a serious medical condition, which could leave him paralyzed for life. Brad, on the other hand, did not seem as upset as you'd think he should be, under the circumstances.

On the evening of admission things began to quiet down and the pediatric resident on duty was able to spend some extra time with Brad. They talked very openly with each other, and the resident soon realized that the boy was having a hard time with some teens his own age. The resident gently kept asking questions about this topic, and discovered that there was a bully on the school bus who was threatening Brad. Brad feared for his safety because the other boy was much bigger and stronger. Brad also was afraid that he would be beaten up if he told anyone about this.

It soon became obvious to the resident that Brad was suffering from what is called a 'conversion reaction.' This type of emotional response to a mental conflict is fairly common during adolescence. Such reactions may take on many forms including hysterical blindness, seizures, gait (walking) disturbances, and paralysis, as in Brad's case. With this condition there is a loss or change of some physical function without any visible physical cause or illness. It is caused by mental and/or emotional conflict, and the person suffering from it usually does not understand what is causing the problem. As in Brad's case, a reaction often begins suddenly, and can be traced back to a particular thing that happened. Usually the symptoms end suddenly, after lasting only a short time.

The resident was able to comfort Brad, and broke the news about the bully to his parents. The boy was very concerned that they would be angry and accuse him of faking the symptoms. Actually, the parents were very relieved when they understood that the paralysis was a real manifestation of a psychiatric disturbance. As soon as the problem with the bully was brought out in the open, the parents promised Brad that they would do the right thing to make sure he was safe and protected on the bus and at school. Once he knew the problem had been taken care of, Brad got better quickly and walked out of the hospital the next morning.

Congratulations to the resident for getting the necessary information that led to the correct diagnosis, and a fast recovery.

CHAPTER 8
Birds of a Feather

Friends of the same age are very important during early adolescence. Let's take a peak inside the cockpit to see what the crew may be up to behind the scenes.

Relationships within such close quarters are very intense at this age, and it is not surprising how friendships may suddenly bloom or just as quickly blow apart. As they develop their own inner circle, adolescents need only look over to their peers for approval or acceptance. Bonding between members of the same sex, boys with boys and girls with girls, may be especially strong. They know how to stick together, especially when the going gets tough. Teenagers are experts at learning the value of loyalty, dedication, and devotion to their friends while high in the air on their space flight, and at the same time staying loyal to their family below. Many times teenagers actually keep higher standards of honor and integrity than our society has set for its grownups! Most young adolescents are truly model citizens when it comes to the old fashioned, down-to-earth values that are so badly needed in today's world. They usually rise far above any celebrities, sports stars, politicians, or other grown-ups, who may act as if such moral rules are beneath them.

TEEN TIP - Learning to balance what's important may seem like a bit of a juggling act at times. Sometimes you may feel torn between family and friends. Trust your instincts to help give you a sense for what's right and what's wrong. Then follow your heart to make decisions you won't regret or feel guilty about later on. You'll soon come to realize that you won't be able to make everyone happy all of the time.

Teens who seem to be sitting on the edge of their seats may actually be suffering from high anxiety. Some may even come down with a case of claustrophobia because they feel trapped in the tight cage of the space capsule. It is not unusual for sparks to fly under these circumstances. Problems with friends are a common source of stress and anxiety among adolescents. Usually the troubles end naturally by themselves, and do not lead to ongoing stress. Adolescents are usually able to talk through their problems, patch them up, or ride them out before things get blown up too big.

But conflicts that are not settled, and that go on and on, can have serious results, including harm to self or others. Sometimes a calm older person may need to be called in to settle any disagreements.

Going along with the crowd is standard operating procedure during early puberty. This is a very sensitive period of life, and teens do not want to feel singled out. Although they may want to be their own person, at the same time they want very much to be 'undifferent' and part of the group. Their communication with others and their response to peer pressure is very obvious as they begin to define who they really are.

Sometimes they may do extreme things trying to be accepted. They may act out sexually and sleep with others so they can feel wanted. They may use drugs to comfort themselves and get rid of feelings of not being accepted. They may do high-risk things like speeding in vehicles to be part of the crowd. They may do unhealthy things to improve their appearance, like starve themselves to be thin. So it is very important for the ground crew to continue to keep tabs on their children before things get too far out of hand.

This may be no easy task - part of the excitement and adventure for many adolescents is keeping their parents in the dark. It may be difficult for some parents to accept that they are no longer their teen's best friend, when up until the beginning of adolescence they have always shared everything with each other. This is an especially tough time for mothers who once felt so close to their daughters and now feel as though they are drifting apart. In reality, their teenager is growing up and developing a sense of independence that is actually a very healthy sign. Parents should expect that as adolescents grow up they will be more apt to share secrets with their friends, and no longer always confide in their parents.

PARENT TIP - If you feel left out of the loop, do not despair. This is all part of the separation process, and does not mean you're doing a poor job of being a parent. As difficult as it may seem, parents who accept this as a normal phase of adolescent development will be rewarded for their patience and understanding when maturation is complete. Words can not describe how wonderful it feels to be able to carry on a civil conversation once again as your son or daughter finally reaches adulthood. In contrast, parents who still insist on knowing everything or being too nosey may actually endanger the mission by not giving their teenager enough space to grow.

Don't smother me

Tara was a 14-year-old girl referred to me for her behavior problems at home as well as at school. She would frequently argue with her mother because she believed her mother was nosey and overprotective. The two would often fight about Tara skipping school, and her falling grades. The girl had also made a secret vow with one of her friends to begin vomiting, to try to lose weight. Tara lost about eight pounds in a few weeks, but she told me that over the past two months her weight had stayed the same when she stopped throwing up. Tara was also having problems with a boyfriend her mother did not like. Her mother stated she was 'at wit's end.' She felt her daughter was spinning out of control, and she was in the process of filing a PINS (person in need of supervision) petition against her. To make things even more complicated, the mother was trying to raise Tara by herself because the father was an alcoholic and had not been in the family for a long time.

The situation at home was so serious that the mother was worried that someone was going to get hurt. Tara had overdosed on aspirin earlier that year after another argument with her mother. Tara told me that she had done this more out of anger, and that she did not really want to hurt herself. She also had scars over her forearms from cutting herself with a knife several months earlier. Things were not going well for Tara at school and she was skipping school regularly. Her peer supports were also falling apart, after she had had many arguments and numerous verbal confrontations with her best friends. She had a physical fight with her boyfriend, and she was injured when he struck her in the chest. She would often take out her frustrations by yelling at her mother or throwing things around the house. One time she broke several dishes and accidentally cut herself in the process. Life was not good for Tara.

Things only seemed to get worse. After a 'bad conversation' with her boyfriend over the phone, Tara wanted to kill herself. She required immediate psychiatric intervention and was hospitalized in an inpatient psychiatric facility for several days. After she was released Tara still did not want to follow her mother's rules. She was still seeing her boyfriend, but did not tell her mother. Tara would often spend the night at a friend's house and have unprotected sex.

Once her mother got wind of this she went ahead and filed the PINS petition. By court order Tara was removed from her home and directed to live in a foster home. She spent several days there and gradually came to realize that things weren't quite as bad as she had thought when living with her mother.

The physical separation from her mother seemed to work in this case. This is an excellent method in unstable, dangerous situations, as long as the adolescent has a safe place to go.

Once Tara was reunited with her mother the atmosphere became much calmer. Under the guidance of a family therapist, she was able to earn more freedom. The mother allowed her to get back together with her boyfriend once she was convinced that he would treat Tara with more respect. The mother also found help for her daughter in dealing with sex, and agreed with Tara's decision to be placed on birth control pills.

The therapist and I spent a lot of time helping Tara learn how to cope with peer pressure, a major trigger factor for many of her hasty behaviors. Relationships with her friends got better, and she was also able to return to school on a regular basis. As time passed, Tara began to feel better and she finally was able to show her warm, tender side. We knew it was there all along – it was simply buried under all the emotional disturbances.

CHAPTER 9
Society Says

Image is important to young adolescents as they leave the launch pad and become very concerned with how they appear to others, especially of their own age. The pressures to be perfect, or at least to have a perfect image, begin to build up. As they rise through the atmosphere they may be blinded by the unfiltered rays of sunshine and insistent demands of today's society. This may force them to put on a pair of shades, squint, or look away as the separation process goes on. They may even need to pull down their helmet's visor, which has been installed just so they can get more relief or protection.

As they look into the vanity mirror they may get a twisted, unrealistic picture because their eyes are still trying to adjust. The image they see is changing rapidly, and they may not like it very much. Their reactions to that image are heavily swayed by the opinions of peers and they often have no interest in any input from outside parties like their parents or other adults. Many teens are unhappy with their looks or uncomfortable with their appearance. In a study of 854 adolescent girls by D.C. Moore, 67% were unhappy with their weight and 54% were unhappy with their body shape. Corresponding values for the 895 adolescent boys showed that 42% didn't like their weight and 35% didn't like how they looked.

As they lose the protection of childhood, it is painfully obvious that many young adolescents are very susceptible to constant television, movie, and video messages that say you have to look and be perfect to be happy. This often makes teens feel bad about themselves. They may see themselves as failures because they do not measure up to these perfect standards.

Worries about body image and other imaginary defects and imperfections are tough to avoid at this stage. These perceptions are very powerful, and very real to adolescents. Sometimes they may seem like a bad dream or nightmare come true.

Any internal distress signals about looks or appearance must not be ignored by those on guard duty, even though everything seems to check out okay on the surface. Such bad feelings run deep, and something must be done about them before they start to take over the controls. What others see or feel won't change the mind or perceptions of teens who are already functioning on autopilot. The main rule here is to acknowledge any mistaken perceptions as they *truly* exist in the eyes of the adolescent, and then do something to help correct that perception. Sometimes advice from a health care professional is needed so the teen can be brought back to reality, reprogrammed, and shown how to regain control of his or her life.

It must also be pointed out that feelings of low self-esteem and poor body image often correlate with suicidal thoughts, substance abuse, sexual acting-out, pregnancy, and other risk-taking behaviors.

Putting the finger on the pain

Sometimes it's not the adolescent who's having problems seeing things properly. Jake was a 13-year-old boy referred to me for treatment of anorexia and a 20-pound weight loss. He had been healthy until six weeks before I saw him, which was when he developed sharp pain in the right lower abdomen after he had been squeezed in a bear hug during a wrestling match. The pain wouldn't go away, and when Jake's pediatrician evaluated him, he felt Jake should go into the hospital.

A very thorough exam did not find any physical reason for Jake's pain, and he was told that his suffering was 'all in his head.' Jake became very upset over this claim, and immediately told everyone that he was not going to eat or drink until the cause of the pain was found.

He was fed intravenously with IVs. After his hunger strike went on for a few days he was transferred to me, because the doctors thought he had an eating disorder.

He kept complaining of pinpoint pain that would not go away, in the same location in the right lower abdomen. This area was also very tender to the touch. Even when he was distracted and looking the other way the pain remained in exactly the same place.

He also had a small physical defect in the same place where he was tender. It turned out to be what is called a *Spigelian hernia*, which is a type of defect in the abdominal wall. It was probably made worse by the bear hug he got while wrestling.

The hernia was easily fixed with surgery, and the pain disappeared immediately. But it took more than two years for Jake to recover emotionally from being told that the pain was all in his head.

It is very sad when an adolescent with unexplained weight loss is told he or she has an eating disorder, just because all the medical tests don't find a cause, and no other reason seems to fit. One of the main rules in medicine is that mental explanations for physical problems should be made only when specific criteria are met, not when physical causes can't be found. Patients who really do have anorexia have a twisted idea of what their body looks like, a fear of being fat, a strong desire to lose weight, and they will not eat fatty foods. Jake had none of these symptoms. Also, his symptom of pinpoint pain that would not go away, and tenderness on exam in the same location, should be considered to have a physical origin until proven otherwise. While Jake did not actually have body image concerns, his story is included in this section so that other adolescents with unexplained weight loss will not meet with a similar misfortune and suffer unnecessarily as he did.

★★★★★★

Young adolescents may want a complete makeover as they leave the launch pad and get the message that image *is* everything. They constantly think about themselves, and the physical changes that are taking place. This may cause uncertainty as their development moves along, and they fear they might fall short of the mark. While such thoughts are quite normal and natural, they are easily blown out of proportion in our society, which insists on perfection. It's no wonder our teens are so often down in the dumps about how they look. After all, they are growing up in a world where they see adults getting facelifts, breast implants, nose jobs, and tummy tucks to improve their looks. Unwanted body hair can be dissolved in a flash. Even fat deposits can be gotten rid of by a surgeon's scalpel or suction equipment. There's nothing wrong with wanting to look good, but it gets a little messy when adolescents who want to look perfect wind up getting stuck on themselves.

For those desperate to have greater muscle bulk, power, or speed, it may take real strength to set the record straight. Although performance-enhancing drugs have been around for some time, they have received a lot of publicity during the past several years. Professionals and other high profile athletes can decide for themselves if use of such drugs is worth the possible bad results to their health or their reputation. This is their business. It's my business to raise public awareness, so adolescents do not fall victim to society's pressures to be perfect, or imitate heroes who may use potentially harmful drugs.

PARENT TIP - It's very tempting for young competitors to follow the example of sports stars who use performance - enhancing drugs to gain a competitive edge. However, such practices by professional athletes set a potentially dangerous example for today's youth. Talk to your teenager about the fact that the safety of these drugs has not yet been clearly established, and there are particular concerns that they may cause serious side effects in adolescents as well as younger children.

Of particular concern is the wrong message that has been sent to so many youngsters who look up to sports stars and want to follow in their footsteps. They're already beating down a path to health food stores and other suppliers. Many of the controversial performance-enhancing substances are available over the counter, and are as easy to buy as candy. Sales have increased rapidly in spite of the high cost, and there are serious worries that there will be an even greater price paid physically, because of potential side effects.

The illegal black market for more powerful prescription compounds has also grown fast, through the efforts of various unscrupulous individuals, including a small number of doctors, pharmacists, and even coaches. It is obvious that the federal Food and Drug Administration (FDA) needs to get a better grip, and control these drugs in an effort to keep them off the street and out of the hands of adolescents. Leading athletic organizations also have a public obligation to actively speak out against the use of performance enhancing drugs, and should not merely provide lip service when doing so. Finally, sports stars who have relied on power building pills, powders, and shots can still clean up their act and save face in the public's eye. Maybe they all should call a press conference and flush the products down the drain on the count of three. I can just hear that giant gurgling sound right now. That would definitely get the attention of their adolescent followers. After all, actions speak louder than words to young admiring fans.

Making a statement with tattoos and other forms of body art is also getting more popular among young people. It seems like open season these days, and any spot of skin appears to be fair game. Nothing is safe anymore from being stabbed, speared, or even shot with an ink gun. Little shops and pagodas where anyone can get painted up, pierced, or punctured on the spur of the moment are showing up all over the place. Teenagers, who often act on a whim, frequently go to these. It's no wonder so many parents worry that today's generation won't be able to hold any water - rings and things can be seen protruding from almost every available opening, natural or otherwise. Some may be out in the open and in plain sight for all to see. It may take a little effort to find those stuck in the tongue or bundled up in the belly button. Others may be buried in secret hiding places which are off limits to the general public, and only open for special viewing by that certain someone. Three-dimensional tattoos under the skin are also beginning to surface, with teens bragging about who has the biggest or most beautiful bumps. Carving, branding, and scarification are even managing to make their mark.

TEEN TIP – If you are thinking about getting a tattoo or piercing, be sure to check out the studio and interview the artist first. No matter what type of body art is performed, it should be done in clean surroundings by a qualified individual who is committed to the highest health and safety standards. Dirty or unsterilized instruments carry a risk of infection with HIV, hepatitis B, and other nasty bugs. Temporary tattoos using stickers, markers, henna, or similar surface agents greatly reduce this risk and may also serve as a good test run for more permanent measures.

CHAPTER 10

Fun and Games

R ecreation, with some time for rest and relaxation, should be planned into the program for all 10- to 14-year-olds. It's always interesting to talk to young adolescents about what they do for fun and how they spend their spare time. As they are about to leave the launch pad, many will put in a request for portable devices that can be packed on board and stowed for easy access. Compact discs and digital audio players have joined the boom box as the most popular entertainment items requested. Sometimes teens get a little carried away and pump up the volume to notches unknown. It's no wonder so many kids are hard of hearing, because their ear bones are vibrating so fast that their auditory nerve fibers may begin to burn out. This should not be confused with selective deafness, which is when teens hear only what they want to hear and tune out everything else.

TEEN TIP - Headphones may seem to serve a dual purpose by transmitting desirable music in, while at the same time being earmuffs to keep unwanted sounds out. However, they were designed as a listening device, not as ear protection. Cyclists should not wear a headset, headphone, or any listening device other than a hearing aid while riding. Wearing a headset blocks out important sounds and noises needed to detect the presence of cars or other traffic. You should also be aware of the fact that turning up the volume of the headphone too high can cause hearing damage if unsafe levels are reached. Permanent hearing loss can happen in such situations, as well as with other exposure to loud sounds, especially when repeated for long periods of time.

The need for amusement must be balanced with an awareness that too much of a good thing can lead to unhealthy habits over time. This is particularly true for passive visual activities such as watching television shows or videotapes. These have created a whole new breed of couch potato. Teens' bodies and brains begin to vegetate because the many shows with tasteless content don't require any physical or mental activity to watch. When adults use TV as a cheap, easy babysitter, teens pay a heavy price further down the line. There is a growing worry that those who are fed and entertained mostly by the tube are being turned into a bunch of deadbeats with no ambition, weak personal relationships, and detached thinking. They will be so saturated with society's sludge that they will not be able to stand on their own two feet and think for themselves. The hours spent playing video and computer games are also beginning to take their toll on our youth. These types of entertainment can suck the strength from teenagers who have far more important work to do. In contrast, as the launch phase proceeds, there are all kinds of opportunities for more valuable uses of the computer to help develop healthy, growing minds.

A dirt bike to the rescue

Ethan was a 12-year-old boy referred to me for unexplained tiredness. He had been in his usual state of good health until a few months before, when he suddenly began to require much more sleep than usual to carry out his daily activities. He was also having trouble paying attention in class. His exhaustion became so bad that he could no longer go to school and needed to be tutored at home.

Ethan had had very extensive testing by the referring doctor and our infectious disease consultants before I saw him. None of the tests showed anything besides the fact that he had had mononucleosis at some unknown time in the past. One doctor was worried about Ethan's downcast appearance, and felt that he might be emotionally depressed.

I did a thorough exam and ordered more tests to be sure that nothing had been overlooked. Ethan was a quiet kid, and it was difficult to get him to talk. As part of my routine questioning I asked him what he did for fun. His eyes immediately lit up and he told me about his love for riding dirt bikes. When I told him about the racing bike I had just gotten for my birthday, our conversation was off and running. He was able to carry on an excited discussion until we started to talk about school. At that point he immediately shut down. His mom told me that she was having the same problems talking to him at home, and that he was also arguing more with her. Whenever she asked him if he felt good enough to go to school he would shout back at her, "No, I don't want to go!"

Once I was able to connect with Ethan it didn't take long to figure out what was going on. He was very depressed, and having a hard time dealing with a number of important issues. His father had dropped out of the picture when he was a very young child, and his mother was working hard to keep the family afloat. She had high expectations for Ethan and would not tolerate any slacking off on his schoolwork. He felt that she was putting too much pressure on him to get high grades, and he started to rebel more out of frustration than anything else. It soon became a power struggle between the two of them at home, and then with the teachers at school. Ethan had a very caring and compassionate guidance counselor who understood how he was suffering. She made special arrangements and carefully selected a tutor who related well to him.

Ethan's mother was working very long hours and she was beginning to feel overwhelmed. It was obvious that she cared for Ethan very much and she was actively seeking advice on how to deal with his behaviors. I explained to her that his extreme sleeping and difficulty paying attention were most likely related to depression. While Ethan was not suicidal he would require very intense treatment as an outpatient until he started to feel better. She partially understood this, but she still believed that his symptoms had a physical basis. Nevertheless, she followed my recommendations and he came in for a number of visits. She agreed to him seeing a psychologist. I started him on an antidepressant medication and kept a close watch on his progress over the phone between office appointments.

As I got to know Ethan better he became much more talkative, especially when the subject was biking. It was obvious that this activity was an important stress reliever for him. He still did not really want to meet with the psychologist, but that changed very quickly when he got to play the media games in the psychologist's office. In fact, when I asked Ethan if he enjoyed working with the psychologist he said, "No, I like *playing* with him."

The mother was also very relieved that she was finally getting outside help for him. She mentioned to me that as a single parent she had a tough time raising Ethan, and she wasn't sure how to act when he started to throw his authority around the house. It took several sessions with the therapist and a few weeks for the medication to take effect, but Ethan began to improve dramatically. His mother got the support she needed, and she was able to reestablish control of the household. It was easy to get a foot in the door once we knew of Ethan's interest in dirt bikes and media games. This is a good example of how play activities can be an important outlet and even therapeutic for adolescents, especially those who may be struggling.

★★★★★★

Finding a balance between saving energy and using it can also be a bit of a tough job at this stage. New patterns of physical exercise grow during this period, and teens may start working out. Going to the gym has never been more popular, nor has the use of home exercise equipment, or the demand for personal trainers. Wrestling, kick-boxing, and similar activities are also catching on, especially among teenage girls. Some teens do this on their own, some need a little push, and others like to stay physically inactive. The dream to become a sports star and to make it in the pros is still very much alive for teens who sit on the launch pad and stare at the sky above.

As they take off, many adolescents feel as if they will become the most talented teen in the universe. This can be a trap for those who have high hopes and ambitions, but do not have a backup plan. This is especially true for poorer teens, who are often given the false idea that sports may be the only economic way out. When they put all their eggs in one basket they are set up for what may be one more failure, because in the real world only a chosen few are able to succeed along this path. It is particularly important for this group of adolescents to have several other opportunities ready, so if one falls through they will be able to try another one. In short, they need more structure and support to stand their ground in a society where the system is stacked against them.

In this winner-take-all world, it is no wonder that sportsmanship is going by the wayside. Our society is obsessed with perfection and has no respect for those who finish in second place. The message given to young people is that being No. 1 is all that matters - what you do to get there doesn't count. The examples set by professional athletes have an effect on Little League baseball, Pop Warner football, and other such organizations. Spitting on the umps, shoving the refs, and similar behavior by the superstars is definitely noticed by the youngsters who look up to the stars with adoring eyes. Kids also know that the punishments these stars get for their behavior usually does not amount to much. This conduct must be stopped before it pollutes sports any more than it already has. Sarcastic remarks, swearing, and trash-talking by parents, coaches, and even the kids themselves, are already common these days. Teaching respect for others starts with teaching respect for one's self, and this must begin in the home. To do this, adults in the command center must remain in control and be careful not to blow their cool in the heat of the moment. Nothing works as well as setting a good example.

People who support sports physicals are also making a serious mistake by not paying attention to the most important medical needs of young athletes. This directly affects the 7 million youth that participate in organized sports each year in this country. Most of them are required to have a physical exam before they're allowed to take part in sports. Ideally, with this type of exam any physical problems that might put the athlete at risk of injury, illness, or sudden death can be identified and treated. But there is no proof that the typical sports exam is any better than the standard medical exam done by a qualified primary care practitioner, in recognizing teens who might be at risk while doing sports. It must also be pointed out that by today's standards the sports-oriented exam is actually designed to take a rather superficial look at the teen's physical makeup. It looks only for factors that would have an effect on doing the sport. It is meant to be done in addition to the student athlete's regular health exam, and is not meant to replace it. Unfortunately, parents and teenagers often think that when they have a sports physical they don't need a regular medical checkup. As a result, the sports physical is often the only medical exam that young athletes get for many years. This happens for a number of reasons. Sports physicals are cheaper, and it's easier to find someone to do them, as well as easier to schedule an appointment for one. And of course parents don't understand that a full medical exam is still needed.

PARENT TIP - It must be stressed that whenever the sports physical replaces the routine examination of adolescents it may actually have a negative impact, because important health care priorities for this age group are frequently overlooked or not even addressed. A good question to ask at this point, is whose needs are really being met by such a cursory exam? Certainly not the medical needs of adolescents who are subjected to the sports physical in order to satisfy various legal requirements of schools, organizations and other agencies. As parents, you have the right to speak out and insist that emphasis be placed on meeting the total health care needs of student athletes, rather than simply clearing them for competition, as currently is the case.

In a time when saving money is important for most families, it is very important that we meet the medical needs of adolescents better, and use available resources more effectively. Sports physicals are not cost effective, due to the rarity of risk factors for unsafe sports participation in the teenage population.

To improve efficiency and lower costs, the multi-station method of giving sports physicals was developed. A large group of teens is examined one by one, in each other's presence, by different examiners who each evaluate a separate part of the body. One might check out the heart, another the lungs, and so on. It's like an assembly line. Multi-station sports physicals can process 100 teens in a few hours!

These mass screening exams have many disadvantages that can get in the way of giving complete services to student athletes. The exams are often done in a noisy, hurried environment where there is little privacy or guarantee of confidentiality. The time spent with the athlete is usually brief and often impersonal, making it difficult for the examiner to gain a sense of trust, understanding, and respect with the adolescent. The exams are often performed by sports-oriented people who have little or no training in the primary care needs of adolescents. Continuous care and follow up of problems is easily interrupted with this method, and it is difficult to keep track of any medical concerns that may arise. Although the examiner may have good communication with the school and athletic staff, the more important contact with parents is limited with the multi-station system.

But in spite of its many shortcomings, the sports physical can be a very important part of adolescent health care. Since they have no choice but to have the exam if they want to play sports, student athletes are in a great position to get the best medical supervision. Specific requirements for sports, and guidelines for preventive services, can be easily included in the regular adolescent health exam performed in the doctor's office. Practitioners and teens can become familiar and comfortable with each other, parents can be available, medical care can be followed up to make sure it continues, and one-on-one counseling, if needed, can be offered. These are the major benefits of a sports physical done in a doctor's office. All adolescent athletes should have access to such personal primary care medical treatment, not just to mass screening in makeshift shelters. Lack of time and money and other obstacles should not keep young adults from getting the preventive medical and mental services they need. It's time to close the assembly line, open the door to comprehensive adolescent health care in the doctor's office, and raise the student athlete from the ranks of the medically under-served. Failure to advance the cause of adolescent preventive services is an important missed opportunity.

CHAPTER 11

Their Bodies Grow Faster Than Their Minds

S ex is an important topic during the launch phase because many physical changes, feelings, and experiences all start to kick in at the same time. Body image awareness and self-exploration become very important as adult physical features appear, and teens get the ability to have children and reproductive capacity is achieved. Masturbation, ejaculation, wet dreams, and secondary sexual changes such as genital hair may cause real anxiety unless the A-OK signal is flashed by mission control. Young space voyagers and the adults in mission control must all understand that there is a big variety in the time that these changes happen. This is completely normal. For example, some adolescents may develop beards or breasts at a fairly early age, even before becoming teenagers, while it may not happen to others until several years later. Most take comfort in the fact that they fall somewhere in between, and are happy to be exactly where they are. During this very sensitive period of life, they do not want to be perceived as different from their friends, or to be singled out in any way.

As they begin to make comparisons between each other, any teens that feel like outsiders may become very self-conscious about being the focus of attention, and will do almost anything to blend in with the crowd. Camouflage outfits may be perfect for this, and ways to hide bodily changes, or lack of them, may be used for extra security. For example, young girls who are early bloomers may wear baggy tops, or stoop their shoulders over, to conceal their budding breasts from the stares of any onlookers. Tall boys may try to shrink and hide when a well-meaning person compliments them on their height. Any slowness in growth or sexual development can be a particular problem, and cause real worry. Sometimes the space flight doctor may need to be asked for a health report, and to make sure that everything is going according to plan. In most cases it's usually just a matter of the doctor calming everyone down by letting them know that all systems are still go.

As puberty proceeds, strong inner drives start to crank up and shift the maturing process into high gear. Desires that have been present but mostly unfelt for many years now suddenly power up one right after the other, stirring up the adolescent. Sometimes the pace is so fast that there is little time to pause for any second thoughts. Ejaculations and wet dreams may upset and fluster teens until they realize that such emissions are completely normal in healthy boys. Getting their first period may be the last thing on the minds of young girls, who are usually thinking constantly about things that they find far more interesting. During this growth spurt it is really hard to exercise self-control. The sap has started to run, and spring fever has set in! After such a long dry spell before puberty, a little sex drive can go a long way. As young teens start looking for love, or going into heat, they may need to be sent for a cold shower to help them calm down and come to their senses. Those who seem to be in worse shape than most may need to be packed in a block of ice up to their necks and kept frozen until their brains are finally ripe. An early thaw may spell trouble for adolescents who are not ready or properly prepared. Sometimes it may seem as if there has been a total meltdown.

The importance of coming up with and going over an escape plan so that teens know how to get away from close encounters of a sexual kind must be stressed over and over. Emergency drills should be practiced so they know how to leave a situation early, before they get carried away and lose all control. Adolescents should also be able to fire the ejection seat so they can get out of a hot spot in a hurry before they actually engage in intimate sexual relations.

Even when teenagers seem to be in their right minds, they often get physically up close and personal so that an exchange of body fluids happens before they are able to execute the safety plan or take appropriate precautions. I always remember the words of a young adolescent girl when she described her first sexual experience with a boy. "He spermed me," she said with a somewhat befuddled, confused look on her face that seemed to put it all into perspective.

Sometimes it may seem as if adolescents are flying by the seat of their pants as the controls get stuck on autopilot. Before they know it, they may soon be in over their heads as they begin to go after more intimate sexual relationships. Those who have a tendency to lower their guard or let down their defenses may throw all caution aside and cast their fate to the wind. In the moment of passion, the manual override button can be pressed in a last ditch effort to keep things from getting completely out of hand. Medical experts agree that masturbation is a very useful and important way to prevent unwanted pregnancy and reduce the risk of getting a sexually transmitted disease.

Masturbation is a normal, healthy form of sexual expression that has been the subject of many misunderstandings, rumors, and myths. Masturbation is healthy by nature, but unfortunately it can cause some adolescents to have deep feelings of guilt and shame. This is caused by others, often adults, who tell teens that masturbation is wrong or even disgusting.

process any opposing views and come to their own conclusions on this subject with a clear conscience. In contrast, those who are poorly informed may undergo unnecessary emotional pain and suffering as they struggle to sort out their feelings.

A new remedy for acne

Cynthia was a 13-year-old girl who came in for sexuality counseling. Her mother had just found out that Cynthia recently had an unprotected sexual encounter with a 16- year-old boy. The girl stated that this was her first act of intercourse, and she was very ashamed about it. Both she and her mother were worried that she was pregnant. Cynthia told me that she felt enormous pressure from her friends, who were all 'doing it.'

As it turned out, all of the girls that Cynthia hung out with had beautiful complexions. They told her that if she had sex, she wouldn't get pimples, and her face would be clear, just like theirs. I then asked her if she really believed them, and she answered, "Yes." When I asked why she felt this was true she responded by saying, "None of them have acne." Her mother could only roll her eyes in disbelief.

It was quite obvious that the mother was not pleased with her daughter's early sexual debut. But somehow the mother was still able to maintain her sense of humor, because she pointed out that her daughter's pimples did seem to be getting a little better lately. We all had a good laugh. It didn't last for long, though. Cynthia then informed her mother that she had been to a family planning center and had just started taking birth control pills. This announcement started quite an excited argument, because the mother did not approve of her young daughter getting contraception without parental consent, although she knew it was completely legal. I then stressed to the mother that it was very good that everything was now out in the open. They had come to the right place, as I often serve as both a mediator and medical advisor in such situations. I explained to them that I was not in the business of playing favorites or taking sides. The neutral surroundings were an ideal setting for them to air out their views and to express their feelings without holding back. And they certainly did just that!

Once the dust settled, it was clear that Cynthia was very upset that she had double-crossed her mother. As her eyes began to well up with tears she asked to speak with me alone. I took her into the office, where she started to break down and cry. She said she felt torn between family and friends as she struggled to be accepted and fit in with the crowd. She also had not made the connection that the birth control pills she and her friends were taking most likely cleared up their acne. Up until then she had been convinced that having sex is what did the trick. I couldn't think of a better example to illustrate the concrete thinking of early adolescence, the power of peer pressure, and yet another myth about acne, all rolled into one. Needless to say, this is not necessarily a healthy combination. Fortunately, Cynthia was not pregnant or infected with a sexually transmitted disease. Without any such worries or even a zit, she knew it was time to count her lucky stars.

CHAPTER 12
Off the Wall

Threats of harming themselves or others are often partially hidden at this stage. It is not always easy to tell if teens are simply bored to tears, ready to break down, or even about to blow up. While they are sitting on the launch pad, young adolescents must brace themselves because they are about to be blasted into the outside world by powerful physical and emotional forces. It is understandable that they may be having second thoughts about leaving the cheery confines of childhood and entering the frigid frontier of outer space. After all, who would want to trade in the warm fuzzies for the cold pricklies? Even under ideal conditions it may be difficult for teens to get their act together and take off in a timely fashion.

At this stage any added pressure can strike a sensitive nerve and throw the whole launch out of synch. Given their sometimes volatile nature, young adolescents often react very impulsively in response to what they think is any negative information from outside sources. Someone making a casual, seemingly unimportant remark, or something insignificant happening, can easily hurt the fragile ego of teens, which may begin to crack along the path of least resistance. Sometimes this crack can be easily resealed or repaired. But at other times teenagers may completely fall apart at the seams. Under the right conditions they may even blow a gasket or explode. Unfortunately it's not always possible to predict when these things will happen. That's why it's important to monitor their progress on a continuing basis so that the right help can be given on a moment's notice. This is probably why most parents learn to sleep with one eye open.

We did a survey in our office, and more than half of the adolescents who came in for a routine exam said that they got depressed or upset easily. Over 40% of them thought about running away at times. Not only that, one third of them had had thoughts about harming themselves or others at some point. Fortunately, these thoughts and feelings usually pass quickly and are not actually carried out. Although such threats are fairly common at this age, it should be stressed that they must always be taken very seriously. When an adolescent tells others, either by words or their actions, that they feel alone or left out of the group, this should always be considered a red flag. This is particularly true because teens often act spontaneously and on impulse, especially if they have no one they can talk to about their hidden feelings. This is a very important job for the close friend or confidant that the teen trusts enough to talk to. This person may literally be a lifesaver in such situations.

PARENT TIP - Don't take it personally if your teen does not always open up to you. It is very common for adolescents to feel more comfortable talking to others about various matters at this stage. If you're worried, ask for help from another family member, a friend, or other concerned individual who may be able to help your teen work through the problems before anyone gets hurt.

As they search for their identity, adolescents who feel unwanted or unloved may try other ways to get attention. The Internet is a popular meeting place, and even so-called 'outsiders' may be able to find someone they can share a common bond with. Some do-it-yourself teens may even build their own web sites to get a sense of security, or to find extra support. These connections can give adolescents a world of unlimited opportunities, both good and bad. The rash of recent school shootings are a grim reminder that such opportunities can be tragic.

Those in mission control should be all eyes and ears in an effort to be watchful, while trying not to stick their noses too far into everything teens do. The key is to stay connected. Under the best conditions parents will be able to tell if their children are about to go over the edge or are about to snap, or if they're just singing the blues. In an emergency, support teams can be put together in a hurry and sent to make the scene safe as soon as possible. At other times, search and rescue crews may need to be sent out for those who have already dropped out of the picture. Special forces are sometimes needed to pick up the pieces, put them back together, and help get things working again.

There are good reasons for having such a sensitive warning system and rapid response plan. The cold, hard facts are that every year there are around 5,000 adolescent suicides in the United States. This is only the tip of the iceberg, since it's estimated that there are 50 to 200 suicide attempts for every successful one that results in death. Many of these attempts are made while under the influence of alcohol or other drugs.

Unresolved problems, feelings of sadness, and low self-esteem are often connected to the three leading sources of stress among adolescents: family arguments, relationships with friends that are not going well, and school-related problems. Sometimes work problems, or the lack of a job for teens who have little money, can push teens close to the edge.

What may start out as an innocent remark, or an apparently unimportant happening, can feel like the end of the world to young adolescents. At this stage they are usually very sensitive, easily hurt, and in need of strong support systems. Those who seem to be a little high strung or even a bit huffy may actually be trying try to cover up their hidden insecurity.

This is why it's important to keep an eye on the emotional health of teens all the time, not only to identify any sources of stress, but the best ways of dealing with it as well. An exam by an experienced health care professional may be needed to sort out the signals. Adolescents who are thinking about hurting themselves or others need immediate help from mental health experts, legal authorities, or both. If fire alarms, smoke detectors, or similar safety devices go off, it doesn't take a rocket scientist to figure out that it's time to dial 911.

But these thoughts and feelings are very private, and adolescents are often reluctant to talk about them. This makes it difficult to identify adolescents with these problems, and treat them in time. Sometimes their emotions are so raw, or they have struggled so hard not to feel them, that they couldn't talk about them even if they wanted to. But while it may be very hard for them to spell out their thoughts directly, teens often show faint signs that give hints that there is confusion going on inside. It is also frequently difficult to tell the difference between the normal blue spells and mood swings of adolescence from the more serious, and dangerous, feelings of sadness known as depression. There is no single set diagnostic test for depression, and a number of medical conditions can cause it. Therefore, it must be made clear that a complete, thorough exam by an experienced doctor is absolutely necessary whenever depression or other serious illness is suspected.

Symptoms of depression include a sense of sadness that won't go away, thoughts of death or suicide, self-destructive behavior like cutting oneself, using drugs, etc., and feelings of hopelessness, worthlessness, or pessimism. However, signs of depression in adolescents are often very vague and general, and commonly physical in nature. These symptoms are quite real, although they may have a psychological rather than a physical cause. Teenagers may lose their appetites, or they may actually eat more than usual, causing their weight to fluctuate. An eating disorder can also develop. Sleep patterns may change so that they sleep less or more than usual. Chronic fatigue, lack of energy and relative inactivity are quite common, although adolescents sometimes actually increase the amount of exercise performed. Other physical complaints of depression include dizziness, headaches, chest pain, stomach aches and pain in the joints or muscles.

Other relatively common nonspecific symptoms of depression include irritability, indecisiveness, restlessness and reduced interest in normal activities. School-related problems such as diminished ability to think clearly, difficulty concentrating, falling grades, frequent absences, etc., are frequently seen. Boredom, being unable to enjoy life, and a tendency to withdraw from family members or friends are also important signs. Also, acting-out behavior such as running away, sexual activity, substance abuse, poor safety habits, trouble with the law, etc., are closely related with feelings of unhappiness.

TEEN TIP - If you have been experiencing any such unexplained symptoms you may be depressed and not even realize it. This is nothing to be ashamed of any more than if you had a runny nose or sore throat. However, the effects can be far more serious if you don't get help soon. Talk to your family, a friend, or another person you trust. Most of the time you will feel better simply by getting a load off your mind. If you continue to feel bad, you can always get professional help. Being a teenager can be tough, but we can make it easier.

Saving the day

Kelly was a 14-year-old girl who I saw because she had an eating disorder. She was in her usual state of good health until four months earlier when she began to vomit on purpose after meals. She told me she was throwing up two or more times a day, depending on what she ate. Fatty foods and those with a lot of calories were the ones she vomited most. She would use a toothbrush to make herself throw up. She also used up to one bottle a week of an over-the-counter liquid antacid, which had laxative-like side effects, and made her move her bowels. Kelly told me she had lost about 30 pounds since she began vomiting, and wanted to lose 10 more. She was also exercising more and was using a treadmill to burn off extra calories. The exercise was becoming harder, though, because she was beginning to feel tired and weak.

It was obvious that Kelly was suffering from low self-esteem, and ran herself down in her thoughts. She felt that much of her body was too fat, but was particularly concerned about her lower belly being too big. Kelly also told me that she had been quite unhappy with life in general, and that she recently tried to overdose on painkillers.

I talked to her for a long time about these feelings. Finally I became convinced that she was not actively thinking about suicide, and was in no immediate danger. Also, she told me that if she had any suicidal thoughts she would ask for help before she hurt herself.

She said that she had friends and family members that she felt she could talk to, if she needed to. I felt it was safe to send her home because the correct supportive services were in place, and she had promised to use them if she needed to. But I was still a bit uneasy. There was something different about the way Kelly acted during our talks, but I couldn't put my finger on it.

I saw Kelly a couple more times, and she seemed to be doing all right. By now it was mid-December and we set up the next appointment for after the holidays. When she returned in January, I asked the medical student working with me to talk to her first. I thought this would be a good experience for them both, because Kelly had seemed to enjoy working with students during her previous visits. She had been very open, and willing to discuss her worries with them.

The student visited Kelly and returned in about 20 minutes. He stated that her eating disorder was under much better control. I thought that was great.

The student replied, "That's the good news."

"What's the bad news?" I asked.

He said that Kelly told him that she wanted to kill her mother. She said things were much more stressful at home, and she was quite frustrated with the situation. There were frequent disagreements with her parents, which also made her very angry. Her family doctor had started her on antidepressant medication, but it wasn't helping so she increased the dose to three times that which was prescribed. She did this without telling her doctor. This increased dosage made her more cranky and upset.

The medical student and I then talked to Kelly alone for about half an hour. She spoke very matter-of-factly about planning to stab her mother with a knife. Her face was expressionless, and she showed no guilt as she described the plot. It became very obvious that this was not a passing thought, and that she had very serious intentions. When I asked Kelly where these feelings were coming from she told me that a voice inside her was telling her do this.

At that point it all seemed to fit together. Kelly appeared to be suffering from auditory hallucinations -- she could be psychotic! After thinking about it, I realized that detached, distant look in her eyes was what had bothered me about Kelly all along. She had sometimes responded to questions with a blank stare, and it had almost seemed at times as if I had been looking into the eyes of a robot. Little did I know that I had been looking into the eyes of a would-be killer.

Fortunately, the student was able to obtain the necessary information to make a correct judgement of Kelly's condition. He had the right line of thinking to uncover clues to an illness that had been otherwise hidden. As in Kelly's case, the signs of a psychotic break in adolescents are sometimes very faint, especially in the early stages. Kelly was not raving mad, and she was not high on drugs. She was an otherwise typical teenager who was suffering from very disturbing thoughts which neither she nor anyone else could completely understand. Up to now, even her mother had believed that these threatening remarks were simply idle comments made during their frequent mother-daughter quarrels. Once the mother understood how serious the situation was, she realized that her daughter needed help right away.

I arranged for immediate psychiatric help, and Kelly was admitted to a psychiatric hospital on an emergency basis. She was diagnosed as having an acute reactive psychosis. In adolescents this condition is usually self-limited, and it is believed to be caused by extreme stress. Kelly was placed on a major tranquilizer and received intensive inpatient counseling. She spent several weeks in this facility and then returned to see me early that spring.

At that point Kelly seemed like an entirely different person. She was bright and cheerful, and she had no trouble looking me in the eye when we talked. She answered questions quickly and appropriately. She looked great, and actually had trimmed down a bit by making healthier dietary selections. She was also very proud of the fact that she no longer felt the need to purge, and had stopped vomiting completely. Her mom was also very pleased as well as very thankful.

Later that spring and during the summer I gradually spaced out Kelly's visits to our office because she was making excellent progress. She was eventually weaned off all her medication and remained in complete remission. When I saw her back shortly after school started she was giggly, and bubbling with pride about maintaining her desired weight in a healthy way. Kelly, her mother, and I all agreed that a return visit wasn't needed. I then discharged Kelly to the care of her family doctor and therapist, who would continue to observe her for any setbacks or return of her psychosis. Hats off to the medical student for helping to bring a good ending to what could have been a tragic story!

PART TWO

The Orbit
Middle Adolescence – 15 to 17 Years

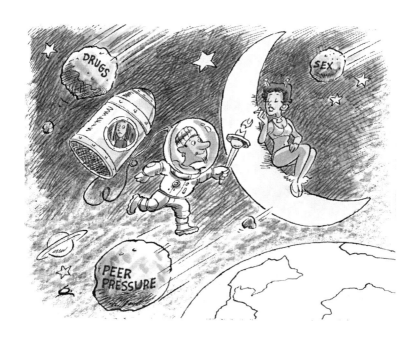

CHAPTER 13

Entering Never-Never Land

As earth is left behind and the upper atmosphere is penetrated, a world of narcissism (self-admiration), fantasy, and magical thinking is entered. The stage of middle adolescence, from 15 to 17, is often referred to as the essence of adolescence. The dream to become a star, around which the rest of the solar system revolves, remains alive until the earth's gravitational forces gently tuck the newly born satellite safely into orbit. From the earth below the astronaut may appear as only a tiny dot, no bigger than a grain of sand. From the opposite view, through the eyes of the astronauts still green behind the ears, flying high is the experience of a lifetime. As they sail above the world in the privacy and protection of the cabin, they now have a whole new perspective from which to operate. There is also a sense of peace and tranquility, because the roar of the rockets has been replaced by the silence and solitude of an outer space retreat. Intellectual capacity, imagination, creativity, and feelings are expanded in range and sensitivity. Interruptions from the ground may be viewed with resentment, and the fear of rejection may limit contacts to safe relationships with friends of the same age. Thoughts and feelings about body image slowly begin to seem more acceptable, since the maturing astronauts have become better at increasing their attractiveness to the opposite sex by using cosmetic changes in their appearance. Suspense begins to build as the search for identity shifts into the fast lane. This creates feelings of being all-powerful, and immortal. Adolescents feel they can do anything, and nothing can hurt them. This leads to frequent detours into the danger zone.

CHAPTER 14

A World Apart

Homebodies they're not. While the act of separating from parents can pull at the heartstrings and create real sadness, it is also during this period that conflicts and fights with parents are at a peak. The orbital phase is an important crossroad for teens. As they reach the point of no return it is a time for self-discovery and soul-searching. It's also a time for high spirits and lofty adventure. It's hard to keep a clear head and maintain a sense of balance under these circumstances. During the process of separation, home may be out of sight and out of mind, but it is still in the heart. While teens march to the beat of a different drummer, inside their hearts the family and people they spent their childhood with carry hidden notes, playing to the same old tune and same old song. This gives a sense of inner strength and security to those who may be out of step, or who may have lost their sense of rhythm.

PARENT TIP - As young adolescents begin to drift, they will often search to the stars as role models for orientation and direction. An essential thing to understand is that activities which seem to be self-serving may actually be attempts at self-centering, as teens try to find out who they are and where they fit in.

At this point, parents and teens may each see the other as completely out of touch. This is a perfectly natural course of events during the separation process. Those on the ground must have faith that the flight crew will learn how to fend for themselves with the supplies and equipment provided. Teens need to learn how to be responsible, experience failure, and even make mistakes as part of the growth process. This is best done under a watchful eye before they are completely on their own in the cold, cruel outside world. But it generally does not help when overprotective parents snoop through prying eyes, or send up spies in the sky. For those in the air, it is more comforting to know that their performance will be adequately monitored by those back home through direct, open channels of communication anchored by trust, support, and unconditional love at all times.

Sometimes one parent can't wait to say to the other, "It's your turn now; you're it." While it really doesn't take a whole village to raise a child, it sure helps to have a tag team with enough stamina to keep up with teens, and to track their progress. After seemingly endless hours of driving teens around, or worrying or arguing over whether they should take the car, how late they should stay out, or who they should go out with, even the most dedicated parents can quickly find themselves exhausted and running on nothing but nervous energy. During peak hours the parents usually need to work closely together, to maintain a sense of control. When one gets worn down the other needs to take over. It is extremely comforting for parents to know that they can count on one another for backup at any time. If they need a break they can reach out and tag their partner "It," and that partner knows they need to give it all they've got. Parents can be especially effective as a team if their parenting styles and strengths work well together, and are consistent.

It is a much tougher job for single parents, who are often spread too thin trying to both work for a living and raise their kids, or for parents who have jobs with demanding work schedules. More employers need to realize that it is good business to offer flexible hours. When employees are treated well like this, most of them feel like they should work harder, and are also more productive.

Finding a little extra time for family activities also adds to an adolescent's sense of worth, and helps keep them on a steady flight course.

A sense of consistency is especially difficult to keep when teens are caught in the middle of custody battles, or have to be shared by parents during their visitation rights. Stepparents, fill-ins, or other substitute adult helpers are especially apt to get the run-around from teens, and have a real tough go of it.

Nevertheless, bringing adolescents down to earth must still be the top priority. During the height of adventure, parents are often ready to push the panic button when they fear their child may be headed down the wrong path, or will never grow up and make it back. The motto "Be Prepared" applies here. Given proper schooling, plenty of supplies, and good survival skills, the young adventurers should be able to put on a backpack and wander off on their own every now and then. This may create high anxiety for those below at home base, especially during any blackout periods when direct communication is completely stopped for a while and parents hear absolutely nothing from their teens. But no one ever promised or guaranteed that fathers and mothers would always have it easy, or needed to be happy campers.

If parents overreact under such conditions, they run the risk of alienating their adolescent, putting the mission in danger, and having their worst fears come true. This may be a good time for parents to take a hike of their own and blow off some steam, before they get too hot under the collar. Otherwise they may get all wound up and start spinning in circles in an effort to release nervous energy. I even know of parents who were in such a frantic state because of their teens' behavior that they literally began to foam at the mouth. No, they didn't have rabies; they were simply so upset that they worked themselves into a frenzy. Needless to say, this is never a pretty sight.

Teenagers who can't deal with family problems may try to solve them by using alcohol or other drugs. They may get involved in sexual activity, and put themselves in danger of getting pregnant(or getting someone pregnant) or getting a venereal disease. They may have low self-esteem and develop unhealthy behaviors to improve their image. They may also use poor safety habits, and put themselves and others in danger of serious injury, or even death. Also, they may talk about, or show by their behavior, feelings of deep sadness and thoughts of self-harm, including suicide. These leading sources of morbidity and mortality among youth are all closely related to how the family is working as a unit. As a doctor, I believe such important issues deserve top attention, and must be explored as part of routine adolescent health care, on a regular basis, to keep everybody involved on track.

Good advice for parents to follow at the height of the orbital phase, and their teens are acting crazy, is, "Hug them, don't hang them." A quick reality check with another adult whose children have successfully made it through adolescence, or a doctor or teacher familiar with teens, can really help parents feel better when they seem to be at the end of their rope. Just when they are about to string up their kids they must realize that pulling the noose too tight may choke off some necessary needs of growing minds. When setting limits, parents need to be clear, consistent, and appropriate to their adolescent's development. Parents must recognize that teens with an adventuresome spirit must be given plenty of slack, with increasing boundaries, if they are to learn how to survive and succeed on their own. There needs to be a delicate balance between freedom and discipline, along with an understanding that the punishment should fit the crime. Teenagers must be held accountable for their actions, yet in most situations they also deserve another chance to get it right. The phrase, "I beg your pardon" comes to mind here, because adolescents need to keep testing and re-testing different situations while they explore new frontiers as part of the growth process.

PARENT TIP - As parents, you need to stay in control and learn to be firm, but fair. Ultimatums should be avoided whenever possible so you will not get boxed in and be forced to back them up. Your teen may sometimes ask, "But, what if I do this?" A good response to this question would be, "There are no what-ifs."

A simple but important thing for parents to remember during those sleepless nights is that adolescents do grow up. *They do come back!* A little time can go a long way in such situations. In fact, the best sleeping pill may be the time capsule, mixed to individual needs, taken as indicated, and refilled when necessary. Sometimes a search party and bloodhounds trained in outer space rescue may need to be sent out to find those who are missing or reluctant to return, but they *still come back*. Occasionally, they may show up at the lost and found desk or first aid station, but they *still come back*. When they return they may seem a little different, but they will still have the same basic markings, identifying features, and distinguishing traits. But they are still the same people. Once in a while a quick look at your teen's dog tag or name bracelet may be necessary. Whether or not they will be claimed is yet another matter.

Keep the faith, baby! That's always a good prescription for adults who seem a bit doubtful it will all work, or who are sure the worst will happen. Patience and determination eventually pay off, and they have withstood the test of time. Parents must also realize that most of the time their teens are not purposefully trying to hurt them, but are simply struggling to find out where they stand. With a little luck and a lot of good upbringing, most mistakes will not be of the serious variety. It is important for teens to experience failure so that they learn how to bounce back from defeat and understand that life still goes on.

TEEN TIP – Failure is a cornerstone of success. If you are afraid to fail, you are afraid to succeed. Just think of how many times you fell down before you learned how to walk.

If their adolescent stumbles or falls, parents must learn how to be patient and forgiving. They should also never underestimate the skill or abilities of their teens to steer their way through problems, or to be properly suited up for a spontaneous walk into space when they need to take one. Given the proper tools, they will have learned how to dig down deep and find what it takes to complete the mission successfully. Tender teens are also tough cookies, and most of the time they will bounce back surprisingly fast.

PARENT TIP – Even during the most trying times during the orbital phase, parents must never take their offspring for granted, abandon them, or give them up for lost. Parents must continue to stand by them and somehow manage to stay connected. Remember, they do come back!

Like good scouts, when adolescents do eventually come back they will have developed basic survival skills. However, they will still need healthy surroundings to be able to do well in the real world. As they whirl in the weightlessness of orbit they seem to sense that it may not always be easy to get their footing back once they touch down on solid ground. They need to know that when they return from their jaunt in space they will have help getting back on their feet, if necessary. Because of the way teens are built emotionally, nothing can replace their knowing that they have the complete, undivided support of a caring, loving family to fill the void and fall back on. Likewise, while adolescents are away, so to speak, they still have a true concern for the health and well being of their loved ones back home. Knowing that every one is okay gives them greater peace of mind and an added sense of security as they wander through the process of growing up. In contrast, significant illness of a family member or friend may put any further development on hold.

Beating the odds

Rhonda was a 15-year-old who came to our office because she had pain in her stomach. The pain was somewhat vague in nature and not confined to any one place of the abdomen. Her exam showed that she was physically completely normal, and all lab studies were negative. I knew Rhonda quite well, and when she came for a return visit it became obvious that she had something on her mind. We then had a good heart-to-heart talk. When I asked what was troubling her, she said she was very worried about her mother. She had recently been diagnosed as having breast cancer, and she was refusing all forms of treatment. Rhonda had a belly full of very mixed emotions, and she was churning on the inside. She was very sad about seeing her mother suffer and go through so much pain. She was also angry that her mother was willing to die and leave Rhonda all alone, because Rhonda had no contact with her father. I met with the mom several times, but it seemed that I was also getting nowhere.

Rhonda came for several follow-up visits, and with a lot of support she was able to hang in there. Her spirits gradually improved, and the stomach pain subsided.

Months passed before I saw Rhonda again. In the meantime she had met a boy, and the two had become very close. She had also become very pregnant. She was actually happy about having a baby, and needed to be referred to an obstetrician. She was also relieved that her mother had finally decided to seek medical treatment, and that she had a good chance of survival.

Unfortunately, just when things seemed to be going a little better for Rhonda, they took another tragic turn for the worse. Although she was not at high risk, her HIV status had changed from negative a year earlier to positive during her routine pregnancy screening. My nurse and I could only shake our heads in frustration. Rhonda's case shows how you don't necessarily need to be at high risk for HIV; sometimes you just need to be unlucky. The bottom line is that even one act of intercourse should be considered a risk factor for this infection. As we have become so painfully aware, bad bugs can be especially clever when it comes to beating the odds.

Rhonda and her mother had been dealt a bad hand, since they both were now suffering from a potentially life-threatening illness. They responded by putting their differences aside and pulling together as a family. The last time I saw them they were able to lean on one another for support, and seemed determined to make the best of an extremely difficult situation.

CHAPTER 15
Testing One, Two, Three

Education takes on a new dimension during the orbital phase. This is a time for free floating ideas, creative thinking, and self-expression. Not everyone should be expected to fit into the mold or perform perfectly up to snuff. The stresses of modern society and recent advances in technology, coupled with the already demanding changes and challenges of adolescence, have created new standards for today's youth. A lot is expected of them. Some high-achieving teens have been given goals that are so high they can barely be reached, or not reached at all. These teens, who only feel good about themselves when they are the best at what they do, are in real danger of being victims of the "Perfect 10 Syndrome." The fear of failing, the desire to perform perfectly, and the need to escape from day-to-day pressures, takes a lot away from such teens' ability to deal with frustration, be independent, or communicate with family and friends. Before we know it, the classrooms will be crawling with quivering robots, afraid to think, speak, or act on their own. They will be able to read digital displays, fasten Velcro laces, and punch calculator buttons, but they will not be able to tell time, tie their shoes, or add and subtract on their own. But with the right guidance, the flight plan can be fine-tuned to help teens realize that progress is more important than perfection. They can be shown how to make good decisions, and how to make up for any mistakes.

No room to breathe

Jenny was a 15-year-old girl who had repeated attacks of difficulty breathing. She had a sense of tightness in the area of her larynx. She was treated in local emergency rooms several times, and sent home each time because the episodes were short, and ended by themselves. She had an extensive medical exam and was diagnosed as having abnormal closure of the vocal cords, which limited her ability to breathe because her airway narrowed.

The exam found no physical or medical reason why this should be happening. She did have a postnasal drip because of allergies, and that may have added to the problem. There was no evidence of a sinus infection.

As part of her exam she was also carefully screened for sources of stress and anxiety in her life. It soon became obvious that she was doing very poorly in school. She felt overwhelmed by all her school work, especially since it was piling up because she had missed so much school when sick.

As she got farther behind, it seemed as if her illness had taken on a life of its own. She felt that she had let her family down, and that even though she was working very hard her academic performance was not up to everyone's expectations. Her two older brothers had excellent grades, and school came very easy for them.

Jenny's guidance counselor was very understanding, and we arranged for Jenny to be on homebound instruction for a few weeks, to try to take some of the pressure off. Jenny was very relieved. She was also seen by a speech pathologist who gave her vocal cord exercises to do, in an effort to stop any more attacks and to give her a sense of control. At the same time Jenny and the other family members got family therapy, while she continued to be under close medical supervision.

Jenny responded extremely well to these things, and the attacks gradually quieted down. She was able to openly admit that she refused to cry or show any emotion in front of other people. She admitted that she usually put on a phony smile, to hide her anger and frustration, and to keep people from knowing what she was thinking. She also described herself as a shy, sensitive person who kept everything inside.

It became obvious that Jenny would often get stressed out, and had been working on emotional overload. Once all circuits became busy, any extra nervous energy would then be carried to the larynx and trigger the attacks of vocal cord closure and difficult breathing. Anxiety is known to trigger physical reactions like this, and they can often be quite severe. Sometimes they can even be life threatening. Fortunately, Jenny had a built-in breaker system, since her body would take over and bypass the vocal cords as soon as she started to pass out. As she became less alert during these attacks she would become more relaxed, and her airway would gradually reopen.

It is absolutely necessary that people suffering from such attacks receive an immediate medical and psychiatric evaluation, to look for any rare organic cause of the symptoms, and to search for hidden stress factors that might trigger them. Fast treatment should then be directed at whatever the cause might be.

★★★★★★

In addition to anxiety, there are many other important physical and mental conditions that can make learning hard. Poor school performance can be the first symptom of problems and diseases like hypothyroidism, depression, neurological abnormalities, decreased visual acuity, impaired hearing, etc. Parents or teachers may not realize that some students' poor school performance might be caused by a learning disability, attention deficit disorder (ADHD), or borderline intellectual functioning. Lack of sleep, being wrapped up in other thoughts, boredom, problems with teachers, and other causes of difficulty concentrating should also be looked at. Poor study habits can also be caused by too much television, media games, the Internet, or computer programs.

TEEN TIP – Learning to balance what's important is always a challenge, especially if you would rather spend more time in the chat room than in the classroom. The trick is to set up a schedule so that you will be able to finish what you need to do and still have enough time for left over for what you want to do. When you do go online, do not give out any personal information to strangers, because there are more and more pedophiles and other predators lurking behind the scenes.

A lot on his mind

Brian was a 16-year-old boy referred to our developmental specialist for attention deficit disorder and hyperactivity, which interfered with learning at school. It was noted on his intake questionnaire that he had lost 50 pounds in nine months. I was asked to see him first, because his physical health was felt to be more of a concern than his academic performance.

When Brian came to the office he openly told me that he was depressed; his only friend had moved away several months before, and he had no one else to talk to. He was still in the 8th grade, and physically much more mature than the other kids in his class. He had a lot of facial and body hair, which made him stand out, and the other students often made fun of how he looked. The fact that he was having a hard time learning just made him more frustrated.

After a thorough examination of Brian, my nurse practitioner and I both agreed with him when he said he was depressed. He was actually a very outgoing kid, and we were able to connect with him immediately. We had him come back for several visits to let him talk about his feelings, and he began to feel better. After one month his appetite picked up and he gained six pounds.

Unfortunately, he also developed a very faint neurological sign in his left leg which had not been there on the exams performed previously. An MRI of his brain showed a tumor pressing on the hypothalamus, which is a regulatory center for appetite. He was given radiation and the tumor was later removed, and the last I heard he was doing okay.

Brian's case shows how important it is to do a complete medical evaluation, and provide close follow-up, for adolescents with serious weight loss. Tumors or other lesions of the brain can not only suppress appetite and cause weight loss, but can also exist along with psychiatric disorders that have the same symptoms. In addition, teens like Brian who are felt to have attention deficit disorder or hyperactivity should also have a thorough medical, psychological, and academic evaluation. These symptoms can be the first sign of a brain tumor or similar physical abnormality. It's rare, but it's serious enough to be well worth checking out.

★★★★★★

It's also important to determine the reasons for any absences from school that can hurt academic achievement. Any severe, long term, or chronic illness can cause the student to miss so much school that special arrangements for learning need to be made. These students may need to be tutored or taught at home. In some cases they literally become homebound, and don't get a chance to socialize and interact with others their own age. Keeping kids at home can also be an easy way out for some parents who don't like the educational system in this country, or who want to have their teen at home for some other reason. Occasionally, parents will encourage teens to miss school to help with the housework, or babysit younger children, or even take part-time jobs so they can make money for the family. School phobia, avoidance, or aversion should also be considered in cases of unexplained absences.

PARENT TIP - A growing pattern of cutting classes, skipping school, or excessive tardiness should alert those in mission control to the possibility that their teenager may be developing a problem with substance abuse. In contrast, adolescents who are having problems at school, at home or with their friends may actually turn to alcohol or other drugs as a coping mechanism.

When the diagnosis of school phobia didn't stand up

Heide was a 16-year-old girl who I saw as a patient because she had been exhausted for over a year, for no obvious reason. Her fatigue was so bad that she could do almost nothing, including go to school. As part of her evaluation by her pediatrician, she was found to have a relatively common inflammatory condition of the thyroid gland, known as *thyroiditis*. This causes the thyroid to work slightly less than normal, which is known to be a cause of fatigue.

She was placed on thyroid medication, and her thyroid hormone level returned to normal. But Heide was still exhausted, so she was referred to me.

I did a very extensive evaluation, especially looking for conditions which can be connected to thyroiditis, such as the adrenal gland not working properly. All tests came back completely normal. As we expected, her psychosocial evaluation showed that she was unhappy about feeling so lousy for so long, and about not being able to go to school.

Heide continued to be very tired. She was seen by a child and adolescent psychiatrist, who found no evidence of any hidden mental illness. She and her family also had several sessions with our family therapy team, to help them cope with this very difficult and disabling condition.

Months passed, and Heide did not seem to be getting any better. Her school doctor called me, and said he was convinced that she was suffering psychologically from a fear of school (school phobia). I really wasn't sure what was going on, and decided to get another opinion from Dr. David Streeten, who was a member of the Department of Internal Medicine at our institution. Dr. Streeten had done much of the pioneering research that connected chronic unexplained fatigue with delayed lowering of the blood pressure after prolonged standing. We decided to test Heide for this condition.

As is strongly recommended, the test was done in our treatment room under carefully controlled conditions. Her blood pressure was measured at 1-minute intervals. After 16 minutes of standing up, she became very lightheaded, turned pale, and began to sweat heavily. Her blood pressure had dropped steeply, from 110/80 one minute earlier to 80/40. We then stopped the test, because this was a dramatic positive response, and she was about to pass out. So much for the school doctor's mistaken guess of school phobia!

The medical term for Heide's fall in blood pressure after prolonged standing is *delayed orthostatic hypotension*. She was treated with standard therapy for this condition, which included extra salt in her diet, drinking at least two liters of fluids per day, and a medicine called fludrocortisone, in an effort to expand her blood volume. She was watched very closely, because there can sometimes be serious side effects from the fludrocortisone, which is a powerful type of steroid medication.

Heide responded to this therapy, but her progress was slower than we expected. She had been ill for almost three years and, understandably, her family was growing desperate. I made several more phone calls and spoke with doctors knowledgeable in the field. After many talks with Heide and her family, Dr. Streeten and I decided to try putting her on birth control pills. This treatment had been used with apparent success in a relatively small number of adolescents, but it was not scientifically proven, and the exact way it worked was unknown in girls with unexplained fatigue. But we all felt that the possible advantages were well worth the small risks.

A few weeks after starting the medication, Heide made a dramatic recovery and began to lead a normal life once again. It soon became obvious that she was not trying to avoid school at all; she simply did not have enough energy to attend. As she got her strength back, she was able to graduate from high school and work at a full time job.

After I treated several patients like Heide I wrote a medical article titled, *Evaluating Adolescents with Fatigue: Ever Get Tired of It?* Any long illness of this type can discourage doctors as well as adolescents and their families. Helping everyone get through such a difficult experience can be very rewarding, but it is not for the faint of heart.

Just ask the coach

Patty was a 15-year-old girl who was sent to me by her school nurse, because Patty had chest pain during exercise. She had a very complete physical exam in our office, and nothing abnormal was found. We did special tests paying close attention to her heart and lungs, but the results were completely negative.

The pediatric resident who saw Patty spent some extra time talking with her parents, and then called the school, because he sensed that a piece of the puzzle was missing. He spoke with Patty's track coach, who was able to provide valuable information.

The coach said that Patty was named after a famous track star, and her parents put a lot of pressure on her to perform at a very high level.

When she was not able to meet their unrealistic hopes she became very upset. According to her coach, Patty would get the chest pain and feel like passing out only when she was behind in a race, and never when she was ahead. The resident then went back to Patty, and the two talked very openly. She was able to admit that she had been under a lot of pressure, and did not want to let anyone down.

It soon became obvious that competing in track was very stressful for Patty, and filled her with anxiety. It was also clear that her parents needed to be more realistic, and understand that there wasn't really much chance that Patty would earn an athletic scholarship to college.

Patty's case is a good reminder that teens who participate in scholastic sports are often under a lot of pressure to perform at a high level in other school-related activities than academics. The pediatric resident had done his homework by making the extra effort to speak with the all of the important players in this medical mystery. If something seems to be missing, sometimes all you need to do is just ask the coach. In this case he certainly turned out to be right on target.

CHAPTER 16

Beyond the Body and the Brain

Abuse can steal the sense of self and strike at the very soul of adolescents. There can be nothing worse than a broken spirit! Bringing a deep, dark secret to light and telling another person about it can be especially hard during the orbital phase, which is a very sensitive period of life. Frightening things that happened in the past as well as abuse that is still going on, keep doing emotional damage. It can be a really tough job to talk these teens down, or to help them become more trusting of others at this stage, when they are so easily hurt. Adolescents who have been abused may use alcohol or other drugs to try to make themselves feel less anxious, to reduce stress, or to hide from reality. Such teens also frequently have feelings of guilt and low self-esteem, or think about hurting themselves. This puts them at increased risk for serious injury, or even death.

Also, teens who have been abused may look for close, intimate relationships, and use sex as a source of comfort or way of dealing with feelings. These adolescents may seek medical help because of pregnancy or sexually transmitted diseases. As a result, there may be many ways for youth who have been abused to get into the health care system. In these cases, taking care of just the immediate medical problem is not enough. Follow-up arrangements should always include ongoing care with a primary care practitioner who can give complete services, and keep a close, regular watch for the issues outlined in the Heads First Checklist.

Carving out the past

Sharon was a 15-year-old girl who I saw in consultation for evaluation of an anxiety disorder. During the interview the girl related that she had been under a lot of stress, and that she was having a hard time sleeping. The muscles of her face also twitched uncontrollably, and these facial tics were now worse than they had been in previous exams. Sharon had been getting psychotherapy and was being treated with medication, but the symptoms were getting worse. During our exam she seemed to be very anxious, and her face kept grimacing and twitching without control. We also saw similar twitching movements of her neck. In addition, she had several well-healed scars over both forearms. The wounds were lines, from one half to one inch wide and three to four inches long.

I asked Sharon what had caused these marks, and she broke down and cried. She told us that she had been raped several months earlier. She said that she carved out tattoos on her arms to get rid of the skin that the rapist had touched, when he forcibly held her down and raped her. She believed that the scars were clean places now, because they were covered with newly grown skin.

Sharon was given more psychiatric help, because it was very obvious that she had many unresolved emotional conflicts because of the attack.

Just when we got the necessary psychiatric help for Sharon, her life took another tragic turn for the worse. Her mother died unexpectedly, and Sharon suddenly had no parents, since her father had been out of the picture for a long time. But somehow she was able to gather enough inner strength to get her through this trying time. Her family doctor and I were both amazed at how calm she was under such difficult circumstances. Strange as it may seem, her facial tics and grimaces, which she had no control over, completely disappeared. It became very obvious that Sharon's tough side was starting to take over and control her more tender emotions. This can be a powerful steadying force, and a very effective coping mechanism under such difficult circumstances. At last contact, Sharon was doing as good as could be expected and about to move out of town to live with relatives. I wasn't as worried about her anymore because I know that she had what it takes to complete the mission successfully – she was a survivor.

★★★★★★

The above case illustrates that cutting, carving, and scarification of the forearms may be due to self-induced injury in adolescent girls who have been the victims of a sexual assault. Self-mutilation is usually a symptom of hidden stress or anxiety. It serves a strange purpose by somehow getting rid of inner tension or turmoil. While they cut themselves, the person usually feels very little pain, or none at all. And the patient usually feels better immediately after the cutting. Although a sense of guilt or feeling of shame often follows, the urge to seek relief this way is sometimes overpowering. In fact, many experts believe that repeated self-wounding is actually a type of addiction.

PARENT TIP – It must be understood that self-mutilating behavior represents an outer sign of inner unresolved conflict. If your teenager is hurting himself or herself intentionally, talk to them about any problems at home, in school, or with friends. Any of these can be a source of anxiety. Always consider the possibility of physical, sexual, and emotional abuse, because they often start such behavior, or add to it.

Children of alcoholics are especially at risk for abusive behavior. They often live in a very confused environment. Many of these teenagers self-mutilate as part of a complicated emotional response that includes very strong fear and anger. In addition to conflict at home, other common things that cause stress or anxiety are troubles with friends or school. Teens who cut and mutilate themselves are also frequently very sad, unhappy, or depressed. An experienced health care professional should examine the young person carefully to see if they're thinking about suicide. If they are, psychiatric help should be given immediately. In most cases, adolescents who self-mutilate are not actively suicidal, even though the fact that they're injuring themselves might make you think so. Self-wounding is usually different from other kinds of self-harm, because it isn't actually done for the mutilation itself, or to seek death. Instead, it's done to relieve personal distress. Fortunately, there's usually a clear difference between patients who want to cause serious harm to themselves, or to die, and those who are trying to get relief or feel better. But it is very important that only an expert should determine this difference.

Differentiation from attention-seeking behavior is also important as it is often felt that teenagers self-mutilate in an effort to get their way. But they don't usually do this on purpose, and may even hide their injuries from others because they're afraid of being found out, or punished. Special attention must be given to the small group of young adults who seem to wound themselves as a way to control or manipulate others. However, it must be understood that many of these teenagers have been physically hurt by others in the past, and so frightened by it that they are frequently not fully aware of the reasons or the results of wounding themselves. Emotional abuse or neglect are also powerful causes of self-injuring. In fact, emotional abuse can be even more disturbing to adolescents than physical or sexual abuse. Of further interest is the fact that some patients are unable to talk about such distressing experiences, even if they want to. Instead, they may express their emotional disturbance by hurting themselves, as an indirect means to get help.

For reasons which are not entirely clear, girls appear to self-mutilate more often than boys. The method of self-injury most frequently reported is cutting of the skin of the extremities, especially the arms. Burning of the skin with cigarettes or open flames is also fairly common. The mutilation is generally repeated, and it's common to find wounds in different stages of healing. A complete physical exam is necessary to rule out injury to other areas, because self-mutilation can involve almost any part of the body.

In addition to anxiety and depression, adolescents who self-mutilate as a sign of abuse often have feelings of guilt, and think very poorly of themselves. They also frequently have a disturbed body image and low self-esteem. This places them at increased risk for other forms of self-destructive behaviors such as eating disorders. Self-mutilation is especially common in bulimics who have been abused in one or more ways. In most instances, the bingeing and purging also provide an immediate sense of relief. However, as with cutting, this relief usually does not last very long, and is quickly followed by the return of any previous symptoms. It is extremely unfortunate that teenagers must resort to such desperate acts to try and heal their deep emotional wounds, especially because any benefits may be so short-lived.

> TEEN TIP - Cutting only hides the pain, it doesn't heal it. It's more than just okay to ask for help if you can not control the urge to self-mutilate. In fact, it is usually necessary. The sooner you admit that you need help and are also ready to accept it, the sooner you will begin to feel better.

Adolescents who have been abused require expert care that is designed to meet their individual needs. Health care professionals must be prepared to take an aggressive, proactive approach to this pressing issue rather than the passive, reactive strategy that has been typically used in the past. To effectively work with cases of self-mutilation like those talked about in this chapter, there should be a commitment to dealing with the hidden psychosocial issues as wells as any medical concerns. Care of the cuts and wounds or other physical injuries is usually straightforward. More focused treatment for adolescents who show signs of self-mutilation should be directed at the hidden causes, whenever possible. Early recognition of these signs and fast evaluation for any causing factors are essential to a successful result. Supportive counseling and psychotherapy are usually necessary. Treatment with antidepressants or medications to relieve anxiety are also frequently helpful.

Doctor No. 35

Breanna was a 16-year-old girl with a 2-year history of abdominal pain. She had kept track of the number of doctors who had seen her for this problem, and announced to me right up front that I was doctor No. 35. I knew right then that this would be no ordinary case.

I performed a very complete evaluation and looked closely at all of the previous medical records, laboratory data, and radiological studies that were available. On exam, Breanna had vague tenderness in the right lower portion of her abdomen. It was also obvious that she was very anxious and under a great deal of stress. I ordered a few tests to add to those that had already been done, but the new results also came back negative. At that point I decided to order a special scan to look for a rare intestinal condition which may cause pain in the location that Breanna described. Bingo! The scan was positive, and Breanna was scheduled for the operating room the next day.

Both she and her parents seemed relieved. I remember thinking to myself that no one else could figure out the problem, but doctor No. 35 had saved the day. Case closed.

Then it was my turn to eat humble pie. At lunchtime the next day I saw the surgeon as he came into the cafeteria. He looked as pale as his white coat. I asked him about Breanna and he looked at me with bewilderment. He said he had examined the intestines several times and found absolutely nothing at surgery. I said to myself, that's impossible because the scan was positive! I was afraid that he had missed it. How was I going to explain this to Breanna and her parents? How would they react?

The answer, as expected, was not good. As I described the surgeon's findings, or lack of findings, to Breanna, she looked me in the eye and asked, "You mean he cut me wide open and didn't find anything?"

Gulp! "Yes," I said. So much for doctor No. 35. Case reopened.

Somehow Breanna and her parents stuck with me. After consultation with another radiologist we ordered a special kidney scan which concentrates material in the urinary tract only. Sure enough, a small, shallow pocket in the bladder 'lit up.' The location exactly matched the area in question on the original scan. As it turns out, the material used in the first scan also concentrates in the urinary tract as well as in the type of intestinal abnormality we were trying to rule out. This is what happened in Breanna's case, and it resulted in a false positive scan that imitated an intestinal abnormality.

A urologist did not feel that the small pocket in the bladder was causing Breanna's symptoms, and no treatment was required for this minor defect. Now that we had figured out what Breanna *didn't* have, we were still left with the question of what *did* she have?

I followed Breanna very closely after she was discharged from the hospital. Several weeks passed, and the symptoms did not go away. She felt terrible, missed a lot of school, and believed that her dream to become a lawyer could no longer come true. She and I had several talks, and it was very clear to me that something was missing.

One Monday morning she called and said she needed to come in right away. I saw her that same morning, and she told me that she had been drinking alcohol whenever she could without her parent's knowledge. She also felt she was addicted to medication containing a barbiturate, which had been prescribed for migraine headaches by one of her many physicians. Breanna said she drank and used the drug when she was sad and alone, to heal her sorrow. She then confessed to me that she had been sexually abused at age eight by another girl, and had never gotten over it or told anyone about it. The missing piece to the puzzle had finally been found.

When I asked Breanna why she did not tell me about this earlier, she said she was too embarrassed to answer 'Yes' to the questions about abuse on the form that she had completed during her first visit to my office. In over 30 years of using these questionnaires, I have found that while most adolescents are able to answer most questions openly most of the time, sometimes they are simply unable to do so. This is especially true of the more sensitive questions, such as those about abuse. Sometimes adolescents are so emotionally wounded by such happenings that they are simply not able to talk about them directly, no matter how hard they try. It is therefore very important to keep the door open when working with teenagers, especially when something seems to be missing. By simply asking about abuse at the initial visit, I had connected with Breanna, enabling her to reveal this vital information when she felt more comfortable doing so at a later date. It was very obvious that the deep emotional wounds she had suffered from were far more painful than her surgical cut or scar.

As her story began to come to the surface, she became quite anxious and had thoughts of suicide. She received immediate psychiatric intervention, and after a brief hospitalization Breanna was able to go home. She did extremely well in follow-up therapy, and the abdominal pain gradually disappeared. A few years later she stopped by the office by to say hello. She gave my nurse and I a big hug of thanks. She was a pre-law student and was keeping up an excellent grade point average. She was also about to fulfill her lifelong dream of becoming a lawyer.

Mission accomplished? We'll see.

CHAPTER 17
Moonshine on their shoulders

Drugs are often used to lighten the load at this stage of the space flight. In their ambitious pursuit of happiness, adolescents who are looking to party while in orbit may find direct exposure to the rays of reality a little too intense. They may seek escape in an oasis where they can cool off and beat the heat. Sometimes they may wander into a speakeasy, smoke shop, or other shady spot for a short rest. Those who are a little bit brassy may howl like hyenas in the lunar light, while those who are a little more bashful may try to hide in the moon shadows. Many do some simple experimentation as they chug a little booze, smoke a few cigarettes, or pass bongs among friends at local hangouts. But such activities may soon grow, because use of these drugs may increase to purchases of more powerful chemicals from total strangers on the streets. Some teens may also use illegal substances in an effort to heal emotional wounds. A more desperate search for a fast fix, and a desire to change reality, may wind up at the dope peddler's doorstep, where serious drugs that disintegrate the mind are easily available and eagerly given to those who are becoming addicted. Dope dealers *want* you to be hooked. Addicts are their guaranteed customers.

TEEN TIP - If you are using tobacco, alcohol or marijuana to feel better, you are actually medicating yourself. Remember, these are 'gateway' drugs. They open the door to a life of pain and suffering, or even addiction. As a doctor, I can not recommend such a prescription for your health and happiness. Then again, the decision is yours, not mine.

Abandoned by the bottle

Trevor was a 17-year-old boy who was ordered to see me by the court, so I could do a chemical dependency evaluation. He had already been sent to two different residential treatment facilities for problems related to use of alcohol, marijuana, and LSD. After he was released from both programs he would quickly begin using again. He was getting into trouble with these drugs frequently when I first saw him. He told me that he did not want to continue using, but just could not stop.

Trevor was very unhappy with the way things were going at home because he was always fighting with his mother. He also had a history of *attention deficit hyperactivity disorder* (ADHD), with difficulty learning. He was not being treated for this, and it was no surprise that his grades were suffering. As a result, he said that he would often cut classes and hang out with friends who were also using drugs and alcohol. Trevor told us that he was becoming more depressed, although he was not actively thinking about suicide at the time. There was no question that he was really struggling and in need of help, but he did not know how to go about getting it.

When I spoke with Trevor's mom it was easy to see that she had many problems of her own. She and Trevor's father had been separated for several years. They both had a history of heavy alcohol use, and had also used a number of recreational drugs. Trevor's behavior was a constant source of trouble with his mother, who felt she could no longer control him. He would often come home drunk and be verbally abusive to her. When she tried to discipline him, Trevor would drink even more. His mother said that she had no one to turn to. As she struggled with her own issues she was no longer able to give Trevor her undivided attention. She told me that she was completely exhausted.

As Trevor drank more and more, he and his mother were growing farther apart. He felt unwanted and unloved. He also believed that she was abandoning him. What he didn't realize was that his mother was completely burnt out, and that in reality he was being abandoned by the bottle, because she could no longer handle his drinking.

Much to her credit, Trevor's mother didn't give up on him. She made arrangements for him to stay with another family in the neighborhood while she still kept legal custody. Trevor agreed to give it a try, although it was clear that he had to play by the rules of the house.

To no one's surprise, Trevor immediately tested the limits of his new home. He soon found out that the family was very caring and compassionate, but also very firm about following the rules. His new 'mom' was also very good about insisting that Trevor keep all of his medical and psychologist appointments. She also made sure that he took the medication for his attention deficit disorder before he went to school each day. He was immediately able to concentrate better and focus on his schoolwork.

This is a typical response for teens who are correctly diagnosed with attention deficit disorder and placed on the correct therapy. The medication helps them calm down and stay on task so that they will perform more to their ability. When this happens they are less likely to be made fun of by their peers, and also less likely to turn to drugs to bury their troubles, or to boost their self-esteem.

Slowly but surely, things began to fall into place for Trevor. He realized that there were people who really cared about him, and in turn he began to feel better about himself. His grades started to come up and he was able to graduate on time with his classmates. The last time I heard from him, he was going to a local community college and also had a part time job. This was no small accomplishment for a young man who could have just as easily been left wandering the streets.

PARENT TIP - As in Trevor's case, adolescents with unrecognized or poorly treated attention deficit hyperactivity disorder, or ADHD, are at increased risk for substance abuse and other risk-taking behaviors to boost their self-esteem. ADHD is characterized by inattention, excessive activity, and impulsivity. The key to understanding ADHD in adolescents is knowing that there are two basic types of attention. Affected teenagers are able to pay attention during activities with immediate rewards (such as media games), but they are unable to pay attention during activities with delayed rewards (such as school). There is no question that ADHD is often over-diagnosed, and many adolescents are being overmedicated. On the other hand, many teenagers are being under-diagnosed as well. If you believe your teen has ADHD, be sure he or she gets tested and treated as needed. When ADHD is properly diagnosed, appropriate medication and behavioral therapy can literally turn your adolescent's life around.

CHAPTER 18
Learning Street Smarts

S afety may be Job One at this stage, but many adolescents are still unemployed. While the external rockets may be turned down as adolescents enter orbit, their basic desire to take risks and seek thrills is just getting cranked up during this period. As these strong emotions begin to peak, the time-honored practice of learning to drive adds a whole new dimension to this already dangerous process. Although it may be convenient to have parents as personal chauffeurs, most teenagers would rather get behind the wheel themselves. A quick fix is the learner's permit, which as a temporary pass may try the patience of both pupil and teacher alike. Taking the road test may be a terrible obstacle to some teens, while it is a simple, easy job to others. Getting the license itself unlocks the door to unlimited opportunities, both good and bad. When it's time to hand teens the keys so they can go for a drive alone, completely by themselves, some may turn their thrill-seeking behavior up a notch and search for high adventure at the next level.

'Accident prone' is too weak a term for this age group. Although it may seem like a dream come true to them, the kid and the car are not exactly a match made in heaven. From the point of view of where they are on their journey to adulthood, the timing is poor and temptations are often too great during the orbital phase. As we all know, even the most practical, well thought out flight plans can go wrong. Excited, enthusiastic cruises into space are not without risk, particularly when drugs and alcohol are involved. Automobile accidents have risen to the top of the mortality charts for

American youth. Each year there are approximately 15,000 deaths from motor vehicle-related injuries in this age group. Alcohol and other psychoactive drugs are factors in many of these fatalities.

TEEN TIP - Too many teens are dying for a drink. Set up a survival plan so that this will not happen to you. Staying off drugs and keeping sober should always be the top priority. Whenever possible, plan ahead so that you do not find yourself in a compromising situation. It is always difficult if your friends are using alcohol or other drugs and you want to do the same. Sometimes you may even buckle under the pressure. As a backup, be sure you have someone to call to come pick you up any time of the day or night, if necessary. Whatever you do, *don't* get behind the wheel if you're under the influence, or hop in the passenger seat if the driver is.

The typical teenage driving scene is sometimes reminiscent of riding bumper cars around a little rink at the local fun park. More energetic youth may try drag racing or other contests of speed as they turn the highways into their own personal racetrack. They seem to take comfort in the fact that the pit crew lies in wait to pick up the pieces, perform any minor repairs, or simply to put more fuel in the tank as needed. Although the injury and death statistics are sobering, it is fortunate that most accidents are minor fender benders with small or no injuries. So many cars with young drivers get dinged up and dented that there is a constant jingle in the cash registers of local collision shops. While adolescents and their parents hassle about who will pay the deductible, it's a good thing that insurance companies have deep pockets to cover the difference.

Punched out

Lindsey was a 15-year-old girl hospitalized for unexplained stomach pain that had been going on for two weeks. She had undergone very complete testing as an outpatient, but the reason for her problem remained hidden. The medical student working with Lindsey performed a thorough admitting history and physical examination, just as he had been taught. When he asked her if she had any concerns about her personal safety, she began to break down and cry.

Lindsey had been having frequent arguments and fights with others her age, who were constantly harassing her. She had been punched in the stomach, but was afraid to tell anyone for fear that she would be harmed even worse. Lindsey is not alone. Worries about violence between them and their peers are a major issue for many teenagers today, and it is often very difficult for them to talk openly and directly about such fears. This is where health care professionals can do a lot of good, with strategies to relieve stress and reduce the risk of injury.

Fortunately, Lindsey's physical injuries were not serious. Her emotional wounds, on the other hand, were quite real. The medical student convinced Lindsey of the need to tell her parents about the ongoing threats at school. Although the mother was a bit upset about what was going on, she was even more relieved that her daughter did not have a serious medical condition.

After talking with Lindsey's guidance counselor, the family decided that the best thing to do would be to transfer Lindsey to another school nearby. The girl was immediately relieved, and very thankful to the medical student who was able to read her SOS signals and quickly get the right help for her.

★★★★★★

Worries about personal safety become more important as adolescents are set adrift and begin to go it alone in the outside world. Security at school, in the neighborhood, and on the streets begins to come to the front as a major issue. As they search to the stars for guidance and direction, teens frequently see violence glamorized by Hollywood and the mass media. Many television programs, music videos, and movie productions are based on violence. Many boys and girls carry knives, box cutters, or even guns for self-defense, while others flash these weapons for attention or self-respect. Some will join a clique or gang to gain a sense of identity, or to enhance their image. Fighting with fists is now old fashioned, while battling with bullets has become the rage. As tempers flare, all it takes is a little drink or a dab of drugs to add fuel to the flames. Murders are now a leading cause of death among youth in this country, and many of the 6,000 yearly adolescent murders happen when one or both parties are under the influence of drugs or alcohol. It's not surprising that so many people are wondering if we live in a culture of values, or a culture of violence.

Who is calling the shots these days, anyway? Having firearms in the home is an accident waiting to happen, unless the right precautions are taken. Safeguards should also be taken for BB guns and air rifles, which are not toys, but firearms capable of inflicting serious injuries, such as loss of vision. Occasionally, their tiny missiles penetrate through the eye, causing blindness, and sometimes even into the brain, causing loss of life.

PARENT TIP - Handguns, rifles, shotguns, and similar weapons should always be kept unloaded and locked up, especially if there is someone at home who may be depressed or prone to violence. Individual gunlocks are also recommended. Adolescents who use guns for hunting or target shooting should be mentally fit, physically ready, properly instructed on how to handle the weapon, and required to pass safety courses prior to licensing or use.

CHAPTER 19

Follow the Leader

Friends rule during the orbital phase, as involvement with other kids in the same social group reaches its peak. Most teens hang out in large packs to find safety in numbers at this stage. As they venture out from the command module, they begin to enter very attractive and tempting surroundings. In these situations, it's easy to lose track of the important rules of conduct learned during basic training. During this stage of the space flight, the importance of fitting in with others in their social group reaches an all time high, and a teen can be very strongly influenced by their circle of friends. This is where good upbringing, a strong survival plan, and common sense instincts need to take over. Sometimes a little bit of luck also comes into play. Good intelligence reports are needed to identify teens who are beginning to drift into the danger zone. A search party can then be sent out to rescue them before they or someone else gets hurt.

TEEN TIP - Even good kids sometimes get in with the wrong crowd. It takes a tough teen to turn down a dare or break the group's code to stay out of trouble in such situations. Be honest with yourself. Denying what's going on only complicates this already dangerous process. If it seems like you're getting in over your head, get out now. The farther you go, the more difficult it will be to break away.

It's important that adolescents have someone to talk to in times of need. In general, girls appear more willing than boys to share their innermost concerns with others. Nearly all of the young women in a study in our office said that they had someone they could talk to about anything at all. By comparison, more than one fourth of the boys said they had no such close friend or confidant. These study results suggest that young men may have a harder time talking about their deepest feelings with someone else. The study findings provide actual statistics to support the common belief that girls tend to have better emotional networks than boys. What is not as generally appreciated is that boys do have a soft, tender side, and girls can be plenty tough when necessary. Whatever their make-up or personality, teenagers who are unwilling or unable to build good support systems may have a hard time dealing with stress, anxiety, and depression.

In addition to inner tension and turmoil, unsettled emotional conflicts may cause severe physical problems, or even death. It is important for adolescents to air out their differences and to vent their feelings before they or someone else gets hurt. This is no time for those close to teens to pull back, turn their backs, or give them the cold shoulder. Adolescents are usually very appreciative and very accepting of the kindness, compassion, and caring extended to them by others during the more tender times. Most will grab hold of the lifeline. But those adults on guard duty may need to jump in after a few.

PARENT TIP - Having someone to lean on can be a lifesaver in such situations. This is a vital role for the confidant who may be a family member, a friend, or other trusted person in the teenager's life. Whether they belong to a group, prefer to go it alone, or tend to be more of a homebody, it is important for adolescents to have immediate and direct access to a person with whom they can talk to about *anything at all*. Remember, at this age teenagers do not always voice their innermost concerns to parents, no matter how good their relationship.

Puppy love with power and passion

Gina was a 15-year-old girl I examined because she possibly had an eating disorder. She had been limiting what she ate and had dropped from 110 pounds to 98 pounds over a 3-month period.

There were many other hidden stress factors, and Gina was especially concerned that she was overweight. This had become a major issue for her when one of her friends said she was fat. Gina was very sensitive and took this comment to heart. She was particularly concerned that her stomach was too big, and she had been doing numerous exercises, including tummy crunches, to tone up.

Gina's inner struggles reached the surface when she fainted for no apparent reason on a warm summer day. She got medical attention, and everything checked out okay. She was then referred to me for further evaluation.

It soon became apparent that Gina was a very intense young woman who would do almost anything to fit in with the crowd. She was very possessive of her new boyfriend and wanted him all to herself. Things quickly got out of hand when he went out with another girl. Gina became extremely jealous and simply could not deal with this situation. At that point she felt that she had no one to turn to, and that she wanted to die. She became actively suicidal and cut both wrists as an act of desperation. The cuts were superficial, but it was apparent that the emotional wounds were deep.

Gina spent a few days in a psychiatric hospital and was released once everyone was comfortable that she would be safe. She was followed closely as an outpatient, and developed a good relationship with her therapist. Her boyfriend broke up with her, but she still loved him and missed him dearly. She got a lot of support from her family as she continued to struggle over a period of months. Slowly, but surely, she became more functional and was able to go back to all of her regular activities. She regained an appropriate amount of weight and her eating disorder was under control. Things could have just as easily gone the other way, because she truly did want to die when she cut her wrists.

Gina's story shows how teens often react on impulse when they feel any sense of rejection from peers. Serious consequences and even death may occur under these circumstances. This is especially true when adolescents do not have a close friend, their age or older, with whom they can discuss their innermost problems. Teens who are very private and keep their feelings very much to themselves can be very difficult to read, and others who pick up on any SOS signals should seek help for them immediately.

CHAPTER 20
Food, Fashion and Fitness

Image *is* everything at the high point of the adventure, when adolescents are so self-conscious. They are highly sensitive to society's demands on how they should look, feel and act during this stage of development. Concerns about making their body more attractive reach a new high at a time when risk-taking and acting-out behaviors are also greatly speeded up. The results are not always pretty. To observers on the ground, it may seem as if those in orbit are totally out of touch with reality and beyond any reach or reason. In short it is felt that they are simply impossible. Then again, this is mid-adolescence. It is the teenage equivalent to the 'terrible twos,' and it is the very heart and soul of adolescence. Much like those troublesome toddler years, this should also be just a passing phase. In the meantime, parents may be left mumbling to themselves as they wonder which end is up.

Adolescents may even outguess themselves as they start to spin in circles and begin to doubt how other people see them. Many teens get caught up in the process of trying to look good, as any feedback about their image is magnified, and there are so many distorted messages from others to confuse their thinking. Even if they have been properly instructed and thoroughly protected, their minds are still easily influenced and brainwashed by outside opinions. During this stage and place in orbit, adolescents are quickly attracted to false values, and their sense of who they are is easily stolen as they begin to fall under society's spell.

Magazines, movies, TV, and an army of advertisers are constantly blinding adolescents as they turn up the lights and take aim at this age group. Teens are prime targets for any advertisements that tell them what to eat, what to wear, or what kind of workouts to do. Just look at the magazine rack next to the checkout counter at the local supermarket. Thin is in and fat is out. Most of the cover pages will have the words fat, diet, or weight on them. There is very strong focus on the mid-section of the body. The perfect girl is shown as having a tiny tummy with a slim waist, slender thighs, no hips, and rock hard buns. This is a lot to sandwich into one body, no matter how you slice it.

TEEN TIP - Many teenagers truly believe that they can reshape this or that part of their body any way they want, to meet society's standards. Unfortunately, Mother Nature usually does not cooperate. It's very difficult to change weight in one area and not the others. Toning up, on the other hand, is an achievable and more realistic goal. Repetitive exercises to targeted areas such as sit-ups or crunches for the lower abdomen, may be very helpful in this regard.

Because of today's technology, it's very difficult to protect adolescents from the media. With special feeds for transmitting signals directly into the cockpit, it's simple for cable television, satellite dishes, and the Internet to serve up an instant menu with countless choices for the consumer. Advertisers can now even post their pitch on pop up menus, web pages, and other Internet sites for rapid distribution through cyberspace. Unfortunately, what is often put on the platter for teens is tasteless scraps, stale meals, or perishable values that have spoiled over time. This would make anyone's stomach churn; it's no wonder there are so many youngsters with eating disorders. Taking out the household trash is enough of a chore for teens. They don't need or deserve to be stuffed with society's garbage. Network executives, programmers, and planners who continue to chew their cud and refuse to clean up their act need to be put in the recycle bin and placed out at the curb. Maybe next time around they will get it right and serve a more useful purpose.

With the above as a backdrop, it's not difficult to understand why unprotected adolescents worry about their body image and have low self-esteem. All it takes is an unkind word or unlucky remark to set off their built-in alarms. Sometimes they are the victims of an obvious hit and run attack deliberately meant to hurt them, while at other times there may be no apparent reason why their negative feelings were triggered. Well-intended remarks are often taken the wrong way, taken personally, or seen as negative. It's difficult to keep everything on an even keel at this stage, especially when it comes to adolescent eating patterns. Sometimes what started out as a sensible diet soon sends teens tumbling out of control, and reasonable goals become replaced by irrational thoughts, with no bottom in sight. It's not worth worrying over three squares or between-meal snacks at this point. This is a time to chew the fat with teens, pick up the pieces, and put the broken parts back together.

To get the skinny on eating disorders in adolescents, we must first size up the competition, also known as 'Ed and Eddie.' A psychologist I have worked with shortens the term 'eating disorder' by combining the first letters of these two words, E and D, to spell the male name Ed. The two letters together can also be pronounced as the female name Eddie. For many adolescents with eating disorders, the world revolves around food as a source of power, security, and control. Their life is in complete confusion, and their self-esteem is extremely low. They are stuffed so full of stress, sorrow, and sadness that there is no room for any food or nourishment. They carry a heavy emotional weight, and are forced to carry the extra baggage on what may soon become a very fragile frame. Something has to give, and an extreme fear of fatness seems to draw attention to their condition, although this is not necessarily done on purpose. Things often get so bad they feel that their weight is the only thing left they can control. And yet they can not even control this. It's Ed and Eddie who are really in charge. These two can be very powerful and all consuming, and strip teens of their sense of who they really are.

It must be pointed out that adolescents do not choose to be in this situation, nor are they deliberately trying to hurt their family, any more than if they fell and broke their leg. However, their fractured emotions may not be easily seen as such. Placing blame on these teens is entirely inappropriate, and in most cases it is also counterproductive. In such situations it's very helpful to let go of any anger towards the teen, and instead point the finger at Ed and Eddie. After all, they carry the message for a society that demands perfection, and steals the personalities of today's youth. It is also not fair to send parents on a guilt trip, especially when they begin to feel the pain and realize how deeply their son or daughter is suffering. They may in fact lose their own sense of identity as they worry that their worst fears will come true, and their teen will be forever lost in space. Unconditional love and support from the whole family will give these teens the best chance of a safe return. Sometimes an experienced professional is needed to steer everyone back in the right direction again.

Making her mark

Holly was a 16-year-old girl referred to me because of an eating disorder and severe weight loss. She was limiting what she ate and vomiting after almost every meal. She was 5'2" tall and weighed only 76 pounds. Although her abdomen was completely sunken in, she still felt too fat. In fact, Holly was so wasted that whenever she drank a glass of water she could literally see it fill her stomach. She was so irrational that she even believed the water was actually making her fat, because it made her stomach look round, and feel bloated.

When we talked about this together, she was obviously able to understand that her thinking made no sense. But she could not turn down Ed and Eddie, who had taught her how to throw up whenever she wanted to. Holly had learned how to start the vomiting by forcefully pushing her hands into her upper belly. This was her variation of the Heimlich maneuver, and she had her own personal trademark to show for it. The repeated irritation to her belly caused an area of discoloration the size of her fist in the abdominal wall. I realized how badly she must have been hurting emotionally inside, and there was no question that Holly was a very desperate person. She needed three hospitalizations in a psychiatric facility, two medical admissions, and intensive outpatient care for three years. With strong support from her family Holly was able to recover, graduate from high school, and head off to college. Perhaps her toughest test will be staying happy and healthy.

The tired gland

Vickie was a 17-year-old girl who was referred to me for evaluation and treatment of bulimia. She had a very poor body image and was concerned about being overweight. She had tried many different kinds of diets and exercise, but nothing worked. As she became more discouraged she also got more desperate, and began making herself vomit. This made her feel good at the moment, but it only added to her feelings of guilt and self-disgust over time. At home there was a lot of arguing, especially between Vickie and her father. She got involved in high-risk activities, including unprotected sex and use of street drugs, in an effort to feel wanted. She still didn't seem to fit in with her social group, and became more and more depressed.

During her physical exam I noticed that her thyroid gland was slightly enlarged, and blood tests proved that she had an under-active thyroid. This condition should always be considered in individuals who are having trouble losing weight, and also in those who are depressed, although it is not a common cause of these symptoms.

After treatment with thyroid medication, Vickie began to feel happier and have more energy, and she was also able to lose several pounds. She no longer felt the need to purge, and with the help of our nutritionist she was better able to control her weight with sensible eating. This helped her to deal better with the stressful situation at home, for which she and the family were already receiving counseling. Vickie's case shows how important it is to take a close look for hidden medical conditions in adolescents with symptoms of an eating disorder.

The pregnant bladder

Wendy was a 16-year-old girl who was hospitalized for weight loss, and pain in her right lower abdomen. The pain usually got worse when she urinated. But after extensive laboratory tests and many radiological studies, nothing abnormal was found. The exams and tests paid particular attention to the urinary tract and gynecological structures.

She was also examined by several pediatric and surgical consultants, all of whom had no magic answer. However, several raised the possibility that Wendy had anorexia nervosa, because she seemed to have a dislike of food, and she was a bit thin. The nursing staff and I had similar worries, but something didn't seem to fit because Wendy always complained of the same type of pain in the same place.

This eventually turned out to be an important clue to her diagnosis. Our psychiatrist agreed that the nature of this symptom was not typical of an eating disorder.

In spite of our efforts, not because of them, Wendy started to do a little better and was discharged without anyone knowing exactly what was wrong.

A few weeks later I got a night call from the emergency room. The doctor on duty said that Wendy was back, and that she had a large mass inside her abdomen, almost all the way up to her belly button. It turned out to be her bladder, not her uterus -- she was unable to urinate. She had to be catheterized by inserting a tube into her bladder, and the urine was drained out.

She was evaluated again by urology, neurology, and neurosurgery, who had all seen her when she had been in the hospital before. She had fallen on her tailbone several months earlier, and there had been some concern that she may have damaged the spinal cord or its nerves. No specific injury could be found, but special urodynamic studies discovered that she had a *neurogenic bladder*. With this condition the bladder can't empty properly. Wendy was taught how to insert a tube into her bladder (catheterize herself) to drain the urine, and she was followed as an outpatient.

The exact cause of the neurogenic bladder was never found in Wendy's case, but it became very clear that she did not have an eating disorder, like so many of those who worked with her had believed. Just because someone is losing weight and there is no obvious reason, it is not right to assume that they have an eating disorder. It not only can do emotional harm to the patient and their family, it does not discover the actual problem so it can be treated.

With the right treatment Wendy's pain disappeared, her appetite improved, and she began to gain weight. Over a period of two years she gradually regained total control of her bladder, and was able to urinate when she needed to, without using a catheter. Several years after that she contacted me to let me know she was completely healthy, and to invite me to her wedding. I wasn't able to make it that day, but I was with her in spirit as I pictured her marching down the aisle to the tune of *Here Comes the Bride*.

Wrestling with fear

Chip was a 15-year-old boy who had recently lost 20 pounds. He was a skinny kid to begin with. He was on the high school wrestling team, and there was some pressure for him to lose a few pounds to get down to the next weight class. But Chip carried this out to an extreme. As his weight continued to drop it soon became obvious that he was no longer in control. When he came into the office he looked very thin, and very sad. His hands were bleeding from many deep cracks caused by the combination of excessive, repeated hand washing and the cold, dry winter air. He also had severe acne on his face. Chip was a sorry sight indeed.

Chip was diagnosed as having a form of obsessive-compulsive disorder because he didn't seem to be able to stop washing his hands, and a fear of food connected to this. Fortunately, he had a great family with a kind, nurturing mother, a very supportive father, and understanding siblings. He was placed on medication for the obsessive-compulsive disorder, started on a plan to slowly increase his food consumption, and followed closely as an outpatient. He was also given skin medicine for his hands and face.

It took a little time for Chip to overcome his fears, but with patience and persistence he gradually got better. He got back all the weight he had lost, his pimples cleared up, and his hands were soft and smooth. Best of all, he was happy and once again able to display his wonderful smile. That by itself made everything seem worthwhile.

★★★★★★

Adolescents with eating disorders are masters of intrigue and disguise. With fat as the focus, the bathroom scale becomes a satellite for secrecy, suspicion, and scrutiny, around which the war over weight is waged. It's easy for everyone involved to get caught up in the counting of pounds, calories, and purges. But these are just distracting schemes that draw attention away from the basic issues, which are so cleverly hidden and kept undercover by Ed and Eddie. Very often, teenagers will resort to desperate, even dangerous methods trying to improve their self-esteem or improve their image. As I mentioned before, efforts to lose weight often involve self-destructive behaviors such as starvation, too much exercise, self-induced vomiting and the use of appetite suppressants, diuretics, laxatives, emetics or even enemas. Such activities are fairly common among adolescents, and are another reason why parents should always stay on the lookout. Unfortunately, even the most watchful parents may often be the last to know because teens with eating disorders are very clever at hiding their actions, and able to cover their tracks without leaving a clue.

It's time to bring a sick society to its knees! Ed and Eddie's empire must fall. A strong family is still the best defense, and once again it must become the driving force in today's world. All teenagers still need others to stick around and to stand by them, through thick and thin. While adolescents with eating disorders or similar troubles may seem tough on the surface, they are actually filled with raw, tender emotions on the inside. Healing such wounds can be a slow and very painful process. Self-esteem that has worn down over time can not be rebuilt overnight.

PARENT TIP - Unconditional love, love, and more love is the most important ingredient for success when your teenager is suffering with an eating disorder. This can be a little tricky, since these adolescents should not be allowed to rule the roost or assume the throne. Nevertheless, they need to see, hear, and feel, over and over again, that they are loved by their family.

This should help give teens a sense of security as they buy some time before they find their footing and land on solid ground. It should also help them gather strength as they build up emotions that are strong enough to overthrow Ed and Eddie. These characters are very stubborn and deeply dug in, and will hang on persistently. Although it takes time to complete such a change in power, it is a necessary part of the healing process. In the meantime, a health care professional can be called in to help maintain patience and reestablish order.

It must be stressed that most adolescents with eating disorders do not come from chaotic, dysfunctional families that are totally disengaged, as was previously believed. In reality, most come from good homes with parents who are caring, loving, and connected, but who feel totally frustrated and overwhelmed by their teen's illness. It's not surprising that other problems or worries often develop, because of the difficult circumstances of eating disorders. Gathering the family together in a calm, neutral office surrounding helps to create a more polite, understanding atmosphere, so that any underlying problems or secondary issues that have developed within the family can be effectively worked out. During the later recovery phase, the adolescent-parent separation process may seem like a piece of cake which is welcomed by both parents and teens alike, after such a period of intense suffering.

It's easy for high achievers to overcome themselves, especially in competitive sports. Teens who participate in activities in which either thinness or gaining weight is considered important to success, may be particularly open to controlling their weight in unhealthy ways. Such sports include body building, cheerleading, dancing (especially ballet), distance running, diving, figure skating, gymnastics, horse racing, rowing, swimming, weight-class football, and wrestling. Young wrestlers especially sometimes exercise in sweat suits or saunas, trying to lose water weight quickly. This can be very dangerous or even fatal, especially when combined with laxatives or other purging agents.

When an obsession to be thin replaces a desire to be healthy, physically active young women are also at risk for a group of signs and symptoms known as the 'female athlete triad.' Those with a strong desire to win and a competitive drive are especially prone to this condition. It consists of abnormal eating patterns, absent menstrual periods, and osteoporosis (thinning of the bones). The routine physical examination is an excellent opportunity to look for body image disorders, and to educate teens and their parents about healthy patterns of eating, exercise, and weight control. Measuring skin fold thickness, figuring out the percentage of body fat, and plotting body mass indexes are popular in our culture today. These methods feed the fear of fatness, and have absolutely no medical use or meaning for adolescents, other than for research purposes. These are the instruments of a society obsessed with being perfect. There is no more need to use such tools than there is to count the number of fat cells under a microscope. The information gotten is useless, and sometimes may even get in the way of correct evaluation and management of nutritional disorders.

In contrast to the above, young athletes often pop pills, pump iron, or gulp down powdered drinks to increase muscle mass, to get a competitive edge. Adolescents who feel insecure about their bodies are easily tricked by any advertisements that promise a better body build or improved athletic performance. The use of dietary supplements has been especially popular in recent years. Health food stores keep filling their shelves with these products, but sales have been active and they may be hard to keep in stock. The next step would be to sell them in refreshment stands at local sports arenas. One can just picture those long lines ringing around the stadium.

Use of anabolic steroids to improve appearance and to increase muscle size and strength is also very common, especially among male adolescent athletes. Those who want greater muscle bulk and definition, such as body builders, or who need lots of power, such as weight lifters, shot putters, or football players, are at increased risk for using these substances. Similar concerns also apply to the growing number of young women who participate in such sports, or in activities with similar demands.

In many instances the young athlete is not aware of the possible dangers of anabolic steroids and other performance-enhancing drugs. There is a wide range of physical side effects that have been attributed to these substances. Aggressive behavior, called 'roid rage,' has also been reported as a psychological complication of anabolic steroids. Before we know it, there could be bunch of muscle bound maniacs running all over the place. Even worse, they may begin to rant and rave as they get behind the wheel of a car, and come down with a case of 'road rage.' A regular physical checkup is a great chance for youth to get factual information on performance-enhancing drugs as well as to learn about healthy practices for gaining weight, when it's appropriate.

Bulky and brooding

Rob was a 16-year-old boy who came in for a routine sports physical for wrestling. He had gained quite a bit of weight since his last exam a year earlier. He stated that he had bulked up several months earlier so that he could be a better shot-putter during track season. His mother had no worries about Rob's health except that he had become very moody, and argued a lot more.

His physical exam showed him to be a big, strong, 230-pound kid and who seemed to be healthy. But some of his answers on the personal questionnaire were very disturbing. He was concerned about his temper outbursts, and was very worried that he would not be able to control them. He openly admitted that he had been persuaded to use anabolic steroids over the past year, to increase his muscle bulk to improve his athletic performance.

Rob's outward attitude as a tough guy helped him hide his more sensitive side. He had been very sad and unhappy, with low self-esteem, for quite some time. Using the anabolic steroids protected his ego because it made him more competitive in the shot put. But he also became more depressed, and told me he had active thoughts of hurting himself as well as other people. Such thoughts must always be taken seriously, since this is potentially a very dangerous situation.

To complicate matters even more, guns were kept loaded and unlocked in his home. Needless to say I was very concerned about his state of mind, and decided that immediate psychiatric help was necessary before someone got hurt. Rob was cooperative, and the police did not need to be called. He understood that I was trying to help him, but he still felt somewhat puzzled about why he had such disturbing thoughts.

With treatment Rob made a fairly fast recovery. It was felt that the anabolic steroids he was taking had been causing attacks of 'roid rage.' He had not made this connection, but he was able to successfully get off these drugs once he understood how they appeared to be affecting his mental state. Rob was basically a good kid who had been given some bad advice. It could have cost him or someone else their life. It's a good thing he got a comprehensive physical exam rather than a superficial sports physical.

★★★★★★

Sun addiction among adolescents is another important concern in the image category, especially during the orbital stage. This generation is a new breed of sun worshipers, as proven by the recent rapidly increasing numbers of tanning salons. Many teenagers believe that they must have a suntan to feel healthy and look beautiful. But sun damage builds up over time, and blistering sunburns during adolescence have been connected with an increased risk of skin cancer (*malignant melanoma*) in adulthood. Other risk factors for this rapidly increasing and most serious form of skin cancer include a family history of it, along with fair skin and certain common skin conditions. These include abnormal moles (*dysplastic nevi*), which are often hard to tell apart from the harmless (benign) variety. Also, certain types of birthmarks (*congenital pigmented nevi*) are believed to possibly turn into cancer. So it makes sense to stress sun safety habits with teenagers on a regular basis, particularly in susceptible individuals who should be followed closely by a physician who is knowledgeable about skin cancers.

In addition, the long-term safety of tanning salons has not been scientifically proven at the time of this writing, and their use is not recommended until this issue is clearly resolved.

TEEN TIP - The basic principles of sun safety are as easy as knowing your **ABC**s: A) **A**void the sun from 10 a.m. to 4 p.m. whenever possible; B) **B**lock out the ultraviolet rays using a effective sunscreen with an SPF of 15 or higher; and C) **C**over up with clothing, hat, and sunglasses as needed.

Almost all adolescents in this stage of orbit want badly to be the same as the rest of their social group. While a few teens may pride themselves on being different, most usually do not like to be singled out or have any negative attention focused on them. Common sources of embarrassment include acne, being too big or too small, and pubertal changes like facial hair or body odor. It must be understood that one little zit may seem like the end of the world to some teenagers. Those who are shorter or taller than their peers will often feel uncomfortable as they stand out in a crowd. Adolescents who are overweight are often unfairly picked on and laughed at. Those who are early or late in sexual development may attract extra attention. This is sometimes wanted, sometimes not. As shown by the following case, self-esteem is also very important to the growing number of youth with disabilities and chronic illnesses.

The T-shirt that said it all

Felicia was a nearly 18-year-old girl with severe asthma. She was very short, with a physically immature appearance that made her look like she was 12 or 13 years old.

One day she came to my office wearing a T-shirt that read, "Small People Make Better Lovers." I got her permission to take her picture, and show it to medical audiences. Whenever I show this slide to medical students, resident doctors, and other health care professionals, they are always amazed when they find out how old she actually was. I stress to them that Felicia is making a very important statement. Specifically, she is telling us that, even though she is very short and looks much younger than her actual age, she is still a sexual being. More generally, she is also saying that just because she has severe asthma, which has affected her growth, it does not mean that she does not face the same day-to-day issues that more healthy adolescents do. In fact she does, but she must also deal with the challenges associated with her underlying medical problem as well. Family members, friends, and others who interact with such chronically ill teenagers must realize that they deserve to be treated as a whole person, and not simply identified with their medical condition.

Adolescents whose overall needs are being met are more able to get with the program, follow any treatment plans, and catch hold of any care packages that are sent up from below. Those who are not getting their needs met may actually take out any frustrations or anger toward their illness by denying that they are sick, and doing self-destructive things. I have seen many asthmatics start smoking, diabetics consume enormous amounts of sweets, and epileptics drink large amounts of alcohol, increasing the chance of a seizure. Many such teenagers also do not take their medications as another act of defiance or rebellion.

PARENT TIP – It is especially difficult for teenagers to deal with any chronic condition that threatens their independence, at a time when being in control is of the most importance to them. The orbital phase, or middle adolescence, poses a particular challenge in this regard. The key is to convince these teens that by following the prescribed treatment plan they will be more likely to remain in charge of their life and be able to live it to its potential. Looking at these adolescents as a whole person with the same basic needs and desires as others their age, in addition to taking care of the needs of their illness, will help this process greatly.

CHAPTER 21

Give 'em a Break

Recreation and responsibility go hand in hand. This can be a tough juggling act for adolescents while they whirl around in orbit. It's not always easy for teens to keep what's important straight when they're spinning in circles. They may get a little dizzy during this part of the journey when there are so many projects to finish in a fairly short period of time. As adolescents begin to assume more responsibilities, it's important that they are still able to enjoy some of the good things about being a kid. Before they know it life could pass them by, especially when they're weighed down by heavy burdens back home. Just as with keeping important commitments, taking a break now and then must be considered a high priority. With the right planning, a little rest and relaxation can usually be worked into the program.

TEEN TIP - It takes a little practice to learn how to balance what's important in your life. If you are involved in many activities or have a job, you will need to juggle your schedule so that there will be enough time to complete the most important tasks. This doesn't necessarily mean that homework or household chores must be done first, nor does it does mean that they should be put off, either. Be sure to set aside some free time for yourself each day during the school week, even if it is only a few minutes. Take at least one night off on the weekends, and make the most of it. After all, you deserve it.

Adolescents who are given too many adult responsibilities and who are not given relief from time to time may become what is known as a 'parentified' child. The words, "All work and no play makes Jack a dull boy," apply here. It also makes Jack an empty man if he was robbed of one of life's greatest treasures - childhood. When this happens, a number of body alarms may go off and send distress signals that show themselves as various physical symptoms, or acting-out behavior. It may take an experienced health professional to sort things out or break the code.

Going by the board

Todd was a 16-year-old boy who moved from the New York City metropolitan area to a little town in the north country of Upstate New York. Talking about going from one extreme to another! He and his twin brother lived with his mother in a small house in what he felt was the middle of nowhere.

Todd seemed like he was in another world in more ways than one. He was a very bright, sensitive young man who was having problems getting along with other kids, and getting into frequent arguments with his mother. He was also living in a snow belt area, where there was literally six feet of snow on the ground at the time I was seeing him. We had only two feet of snow in Syracuse, which was just an hour south of where he lived.

His greatest joy in life was to be on his skateboard, and he would ride it whenever he could. This was his main energy and emotional outlet, and what kept him going. He got a bit stir crazy when he was not able to skateboard during the winter, because of all the snow. When he came down to see me in the office he would bring his board with him and proudly show it off to all the staff and everyone in the waiting room. At one visit Todd also brought along a skateboarding magazine in which a letter he had written was published. He was very proud of this.

Once he understood that we were interested in him as a whole person he was able to release some of his frustrations and anger in a healthy way. I had been very concerned that Todd or someone else in his home was going to be seriously injured or even killed, because it was obvious that he had been almost ready to blow up emotionally several times. He also had access to firearms.

To help him ventilate his feelings, we kept in close phone contact between appointments. He trusted me enough to keep it together as we worked through the issues, along with the help of a very talented therapist. After several hard months, spring was finally just around the corner. By listening to Todd when he needed to talk, the therapist and I managed to be Todd's outlet for his frustrations, and help keep him occupied so that he was able to make it through the winter without losing his cool. With the first thaw he was back on his board and pointed in the right direction once again.

★★★★★★

All play and no work is not a healthy situation either. Teens need to be able to strike a happy balance and budget their time as they learn how to meet the many demands on their schedule. Some may need to burn the midnight oil to complete their duties while others may get up at the crack of dawn to fit everything in. Still others may sit back and let things pile up as if they will magically disappear or go away on their own. Those who are a bit crafty may con well-meaning parents into doing their homework for them. Much to everyone's misfortune, teens who keep passing the buck are often still dependent on others, rather than independent, when it's time to head out on their own.

PARENT TIP - Parents should become less and less involved with their adolescent's homework. Sometimes just the opposite occurs. I have even seen parents write college term papers for their kids. Unfortunately, this is not a recommended recipe for success in the outside world. Teens need to be taking full responsibility for their homework by the time they graduate from high school. If they keep sitting in mommy's or daddy's lap they will never be able to stand on their own two feet.

As teenagers continue to circle in orbit, things might get a little fuzzy as they try to keep their goals and priorities in focus. It is difficult to keep a level head when there are so many temptations and distractions pulling in all directions. Exotic activities, extreme games, or exhausting exercise routines are often pursued for the excitement, or just to get into shape. But dramatic changes in entertainment or exercise habits should be looked at with caution, because they might be related to a hidden medical or mental health problem. For example, a sudden sharp slowing down in activity might be the first symptom of a number of problems, such as an under-active thyroid, depression, or kidney disease. On the other hand, too much activity can also be seen with pathological conditions, especially in teens with eating disorders who may already be in a state of emaciation. Sometimes a pit stop in the first aid tent is needed for further inspection, with specific recommendations followed as indicated. Weary parents may also need to pull up a cot alongside their offspring.

CHAPTER 22

Hismones and Hermones

Sexuality concerns shift into high gear as the space shuttle settles into orbit, and teens may feel like they have arrived on cloud nine. They often act as if they are flying on a magic carpet on top of the world. As adolescents begin to go on exploration trips of their own, they may be fairly bored as they mosey and wander through the silence and solitude of outer space. To make things a bit more exciting, they may get a group of fellow space explorers to follow them, or hook up with a few good friends, or find a special person to have as a companion. Moonlight serenades or midnight strolls can break the boredom, make the mission more interesting, and also add to the mystique. Sometimes these meetings can be warm-ups for more romantic encounters, or even a sultry secret rendezvous. At this stage there is little need for foreplay, because the reproductive organs have been conditioned to respond on a moment's notice. What may start out as a few minutes of seclusion can turn even the smallest space or most innocent location into an instant breeding ground. In a pinch, almost any spot will do.

It must also be understood that for some adolescents having sex is like an athletic contest, and keeping score is all part of the bragging rights. Unfortunately, the statistics tallied by teens are hardly anything to crow about.

The reasons for dealing with adolescent sexuality concerns are urgent and compelling. Each year in the United States one in 10 teenage girls becomes pregnant, and almost all of these pregnancies are accidental and unplanned. Of the 1 million pregnancies that occur every year in this age group, there are approximately 500,000 live births, 400,000 deliberate abortions, and 100,000 natural abortions. Over 3 million cases of sexually transmitted diseases (STDs) are also reported among adolescents every year in this country. Chlamydia, gonorrhea, herpes simplex, the human immunodeficiency virus (HIV), and other venereal diseases are readily swapped back and forth in the private atmosphere of orbital experimentation stations. These disease bugs travel in gangs, and take no prisoners. Exposure to one organism represents possible exposure to all of them, including the HIV virus. This is a form of germ warfare with invisible agents that may cause serious illness, and these agents frequently go undercover to operate in an even sneakier way. Infected people often have no obvious symptoms, so they become silent, unrecognized spreaders of disease to others or even a storage place for delayed complications to themselves.

"Bug off, Doc," some teens may think when they are asked sensitive, personal questions about sex. But considering the dangers of unwanted pregnancy and disease, it is very necessary that medical practitioners ask about any possible sexual activity as part of routine adolescent health care. During the personal and confidential history I ask my young adult patients if they have ever had any sexual experiences, and if so what type of experiences. Sometimes a patient may actually say that this is none of my business, but most will agree to answer once I explain to them that I'm not trying to be nosy; it's my professional responsibility to ask these questions. In fact, once they understand the purpose of this type of interview, they usually appreciate it very much.

From the medical point of view it is very important to find out if there has been oral, anal, and/or genital contact, because venereal infections may be spread through any of these points of entry, even though there may be no obvious symptoms. Samples of body fluids should then be obtained from the correct surfaces, and sent to the lab to search for STDs. Teens who have been sexually active should also have their blood tested for syphilis and HIV.

If teens have not been sexually active, they should be encouraged to continue to avoid having sex. Scientifically speaking, *not* doing it is the right thing *to do,* to eliminate the possibility of an unplanned pregnancy, and to prevent the sexual transmission of disease. All other plans, alone or in combination, can only *reduce* the risks rather than get rid of them completely.

But it's still important to have backup plans ready in case the situation gets out of control. We cannot lock up the bugs, the sperm, or the eggs, but we can help bring back responsibility, being careful and picky, and self-respect, by encouraging sensible health practices. Adolescents must obtain the maturity and acquire the wisdom to recognize the difference between an orgasmic, self-limiting perfectionist response and a truly satisfying achievement, which can last a long time.

TEEN TIP - Saving sex should always be the top strategy, because it's safe, it's sure, it's simple and it's smart - very smart.

A commitment to the idea of 'second virginity' can start at any time, when teens who have been sexually active in the past are now having second thoughts and wish to put off any more sexual involvement. Information on other choices for birth control and prevention of disease should be available to adolescents, and utilized as appropriate. The consistent, correct use of condoms should be stressed for teens who are sexually active, although it must be recognized that condoms are never completely safe: It is too common for them to leak, break, or slip off.

It's important to point out that there's no such thing as "safe sex." This catchy phrase actually may do more harm than good. The poor choice of words gives a false sense of safety for adolescents who might try to act responsibly but might still be exposed to sexual diseases whenever there is an unplanned and accidental swapping of body fluids. This happens very often, even when so called 'protection' is used.

Also, all young adults should know about emergency birth control (often called the 'morning after' pill) for use in special situations such as rape, a single unintended sexual act, and broken or leaking condoms.

Finally, if all else fails, maybe we should bring back good old-fashioned, time-honored solutions such as gold chastity belts and steel jockstraps, which can be locked securely in place. If nothing else they might give parents greater peace of mind, and allow them to have a good night's sleep.

PARENT TIP - Talk to your teens about sexuality issues. Explain to them where you stand, and why you feel the way you do. Be available to answer any questions they may have. If you are not comfortable in this role, get them to a knowledgeable person who is. Otherwise, they may get unclear or even possibly dangerous information from less dependable sources on the street.

As they whirl around in orbit, some teens may start to get a little woozy and begin to wonder what's up, when it comes to their gender role. This may be a particularly difficult period for those who are trying to figure out exactly where they stand on their sexual identity. Boys who feel different from other boys and who are not interested in girls, or who are more attracted to boys than to girls, may wonder if they are gay or bisexual. In the same way, girls who feel different from other girls and are not interested in boys, or who are more attracted to girls than to boys, may wonder if they are lesbian or bisexual. Many of these teens have a hard time dealing with such feelings, especially if they have no one with whom they can trust or talk to about their most personal and intimate feelings. They might prefer to go it alone, tell no one, and stay in the closet instead of taking a chance on rejection or even revenge from the public, their personal friends, or even from their parents or other family members. These teens frequently suffer from feelings of guilt, inferiority, and self-disgust. This puts them at serious risk for self-harm or even suicide. These adolescents may also turn to alcohol or other drugs as a source of comfort, or to calm down their powerful emotional conflicts. Other forms of acting-out behavior such as arguing with parents, fighting with peers, trouble with the law, and so forth, may also be signs of unresolved sexual identity conflicts. It is important to recognize adolescents who are having a tough time dealing with these feelings and any confusion they are causing, so that they can be given the right support, good guidance, and well-timed help when needed. Professional help may be occasionally needed in some situations.

Sleepless in search of himself

Luke was a 15-year-old boy who was sent to us because he was exhausted, for no apparent reason. His pediatrician had performed very extensive tests and was unable to find the cause. At the first visit I ordered several additional studies. The results from these also were normal.

When Luke came back to see me, I asked him to answer the questions on the confidential questionnaire. It then became very obvious that he had worries about his sexual identity. When I asked him if he felt that he was gay or bisexual, he sighed heavily and said that he thought he was gay. He was having a very hard time coping with these feelings, and there was no one with whom he felt comfortable talking about his personal, hidden anxieties. He was also running himself down in his thoughts, and the idea of suicide was often on his mind. Luke was not able to sleep at night because he was getting more and more anxious and depressed.

It's no wonder that he was both physically and emotionally exhausted. He was in a sexual identity crisis; he just wasn't sure if he was gay or not. It took some short-term psychiatric work to help him sort out the issues. He really appreciated the help he got, and was greatly relieved to have found someone that he could trust and talk to.

In more severe cases like Luke's, when the teen is having physical symptoms and thinking about suicide, help from a therapist may be needed. But in most cases, some good counseling on sexual identity concerns can be provided in the primary health care setting.

CHAPTER 23
Falling Below Rock Bottom

Threats of murder and interpersonal violence gain increasing importance as teens begin to venture out on their own. In some cases the space shuttle's orbit may fall dangerously low, descending toward a path of self-destruction. On other occasions it may seem as if the shuttle is going too high, overshooting the mark, and will be forever lost in space. Obviously, communication signals must be watched closely and odd, abnormal messages be decoded early so that teens can be headed back on course before they vanish from the radar screen. It may be a bit tricky to sort through the various sights, sounds, and squiggles that are being transmitted as messages back to mission control. Sometimes teens act on the spur of the moment and start to let go of the controls before they are able to gather their senses, or send for help. To the unwary, it may seem like they're just performing a stunt when they start to go into a dive. A sense of panic may follow when it is realized that they're actually beginning to spin out of control. In these emotional situations it takes a steadying hand to help everyone stay calm, cool, and collected. It also takes someone with a special touch, who is not afraid to catch a little static while doing whatever it takes to pull teens out of a spin.

PARENT TIP - Whenever possible, adolescents send SOS signals if they are shook up, or in immediate danger. It must be stressed that cutting wrists, popping pills, and other impulsive acts of self-harm must be seen as a serious call for help rather than just a way to get attention. Failure to understand this important idea, or to recognize that a hidden problem actually exists, can be a serious mistake. Look for professional help immediately in such situations, to settle the crisis safely and to help relieve your teen's inner suffering as soon as possible.

Stress, anxiety, and depression can cause many physical signs and symptoms in adolescents. It's important to understand that these different aches and pains or other symptoms are very real, and may sometimes be really severe. Teenagers and their parents are quick to blame any such problems on a physical cause, and there is a great unwillingness to think they might have an emotional cause. In fact, just the idea that an illness can be psychosomatic (caused by the mind) is very hard for many people to understand. This is especially true because of the stigma and taboos against mental illness that have been passed down from the Dark Ages, and still control people's ideas today. As a society we must be much more accepting of those who are suffering emotionally, and be willing to raise their spirits by getting rid of the prejudice which has been so unfairly put on them. No one should be stripped of their dignity just because they are down in the dumps.

TEEN TIP - No one who is having physical pain likes to be told that the problem is 'all in your head,' and rightfully so. The key point to understand is that the body is connected to the brain, and when one feels sick, so does the other. What might have started out as an emotional illness actually can affect other parts of the body as well. And physical conditions can also be a source of extreme mental suffering, especially if they are unusually harsh, or last a long time.

The deep, dark hole

Judd was a 17-year-old boy who was sent to me because of his lack of energy. His parents and teachers were also concerned that he seemed to be bored with school, seemed to be in a world of his own, and had falling grades.

Judd was a very pleasant, soft-spoken young man who often bowed his head during our interview. His physical exam was otherwise normal and all testing was negative, including thyroid studies. It soon became obvious that he was quite unhappy and suffering from depression. To make things more complicated, both of his parents had a long history of mental illness and were being treated with anti-psychotic medication. They were very down-to-earth, caring and loving people who struggled to function on a daily basis. This added to Judd's sense of hopelessness: He felt that he would grow up with the same problems.

When I asked Judd to describe how he felt, he said, "I feel like I'm falling deeper and deeper into a dark, black hole that doesn't have a bottom." I'll never forget the faraway, distant look in his face as he sat drooped in his chair and muttered these powerful words. This really had impact on me as I realized how lost and lonely someone with depression must feel.

I told Judd that help was on the way, and that he would not be fighting this battle alone. He was placed on anti-depressant medication and given psychiatric help over a long period of time. He gradually got better, and was able to graduate from high school. Better yet, at the last visit to my office he was even able to flash a great grin and crack a few jokes. This was a reward all by itself.

Hopefully Judd's story will show others how it feels to be in the shoes of an adolescent whose life has been dragged down by depression, and how a little extra help can lighten the load.

★★★★★★

Unlike broken bones, broken emotions can not be easily detected by X-rays or any other simple studies. But while hurt emotions can neither be seen nor heard, their presence is very recognizable by those who care and are able to feel the pain. In some cases, it is very difficult for even the most experienced doctors to discover whether the underlying cause of a problem is physical, mental, or both. A complete evaluation which thoroughly explores all possibilities is needed under such circumstances, so the correct treatment can be started as soon as possible. While it may be easy to scratch the surface, it takes a little time and effort to get the inside scoop. If an underlying emotional cause is identified, patience and understanding are needed to uncover the harm and heal the hurt. This process will be greatly speeded up if teenagers understand that it is okay to have these feelings, and they are finally given long overdue permission by society to express such emotions.

Unfortunately, finding good mental health care for youth is almost an art in itself. There are still too many psychotherapists from the old days who work out of fancy little boutiques, and too few who are willing to get their hands dirty or work in the field. Therapists who pick and choose their cases, or who scramble to turn their cheek the other way, along with the very limited mental health services available to adolescents, only add to the problem, especially in today's tough economic times. Those brave souls who have the know-how and who have made the commitment to work with adolescents must be held in the highest regard. But the number of such dedicated individuals is sorrowfully lacking, and access to them is shamefully inadequate. They are also surrounded by many obstacles and financial barriers which block access to care at a time when it is often needed the most. Adolescents who commit suicide don't have the ability to find help for problems that are usually solvable. In fact, suicide is sometimes described as a permanent solution to a temporary problem. It is tragic when teens try to find help and do not meet the requirements for services, or are otherwise denied access to proper care. It is also a sad comment on our society when the system becomes part of the problem rather than part of the solution.

The stiff, unbending codes and rules that run the health care system in this country have an enormous negative impact on access to care, third party reimbursement, and the ability to continue appropriate services, especially for those with mental health needs. Most teenagers with depression do not meet the specific requirements for the diagnosis of this condition, as outlined in various authoritative texts or manuals. In reality, adolescent depression does not play by the rules and criteria are frequently not met before a suicidal act is attempted or even completed. It must be anticipated that teenagers often act impulsively or on the spur of the moment, especially if their cries for help fall on deaf ears. Even when adolescents are able to make important contacts with qualified professionals, managed care companies are quick to use strict rules that block access to care, deny payment of legitimate claims, and discontinue coverage for authorized services too early. It is of no consolation to a grieving family when the inscription on their teen's tombstone reads "Criteria not met."

Is this managed care or managed chaos? Adolescents and their families should not have to beg, bow, or crawl to get necessary services from third party payers or from the mental health community. Philosophically, managed care companies have a worthy goal in promoting prevention and enormous potential for maintaining a healthy population. In practice, however, this concept quickly breaks down when the so-called 'gatekeepers' actually function more as gateclosers, by denying referrals or otherwise depriving their patients of necessary care. If their front line defenses are penetrated, the agencies have many other gofers to badger families in an effort to cut costs, and to further build up their financial position. Health care is big business, which is being driven by the bottom line in a very competitive market within the free enterprise system. But what may seem to have started as a respectable goal may soon become a bad deal for families, because there is almost no accountability to patients enrolled in the various plans. The consumer also has very little input during contract negotiations and even poorer representation with little or no clout thereafter. Thus, many managed care company executives and CEOs with multimillion dollar salaries have been able to line their pockets at the expense of patients whose privileges have been stripped. At present, there is a state of organized chaos within the health care industry as the quality of care is being severely compromised by a corporate mindset known more for it's business savvy than for it's kindness, compassion, or caring.

Nowhere within the health care system is discrimination with a double standard of care more obvious than in the mental health field. With insurance companies leading the charge, patients with mental illnesses are not being treated as equally as patients with physical illnesses. It's a matter of survival of the fittest and no prisoners are taken during the process. As far as emergency mental health care services are concerned, it's time to get out the defibrillator and get the heart beating again. If the medical profession took care of the physical needs of patients in the same way that their mental health needs are being met today, there would be bodies all over the place. As innocent bystanders, teenagers must never be caught in the crossfire. It's time for consumers to flex their muscles, exercise their rights to truly comprehensive medical care of the highest quality, and preserve their freedom of choice concerning the source of care. To accomplish these fundamental and legitimate goals, they may need to hire 'top guns' to join them in combat as they battle with government regulators and engage in dogfights with the health care industry.

★★★★★

In addition to suicide and other acts of self-destruction, the threats of murder and interpersonal violence take on more and more importance as teens begin to venture out on their own. Getting gunned down, stabbed, or otherwise injured are growing worries at this stage in the space flight. Clever and creative defense plans must be worked out with youth, to prepare them on how to prevent outside intruders from penetrating their personal airspace. In an effort to keep unwanted individuals out, adults may need to set up no-fly zones around the home, in the neighborhood, surrounding the school, or at other places where teens regularly gather. But teens must also develop their own skills in avoiding trouble, so that they do not become easy targets or attract the wrong kind of attention. Sometimes they may have to scramble a bit so that unfriendly forces do not 'paint' them on their radar screens or 'lock on' to them in their sights. Joining up with a group of gang-bangers is a glamorous way of getting extra protection as well as finding a sense of family, which may be especially important for adolescents from broken homes. But being a gang member can have other dangers, like drive-by shootings, turf wars, or similar territorial disputes.

The 1 million runaway and homeless youth are in particular danger and are easy prey for any predators on the prowl. Juvenile delinquents, truants, and other drifters may also take a walk on the wild side, or wing their way into socially unsatisfactory hangouts looking for shelter, happiness, or pleasure and gratification. Basic issues often include independence, low self-esteem, frustration, or depression. Poverty is another heavy burden, which adds even more hopelessness for many adolescents.

Careful leadership and direction by responsible adults is especially important during the orbital phase of the flight, to help teens stay on a steady course, learn to how avoid hanging out with the wrong crowd, and keep away from confrontations with roaming renegades. Adolescents who keep spinning out of control should be sent back to the simulator for anxiety testing, training on controlling their impulses, and counseling, in hopes of preventing any future crises.

PART THREE

The Reentry
Late Adolescence – 18 to 21 Years

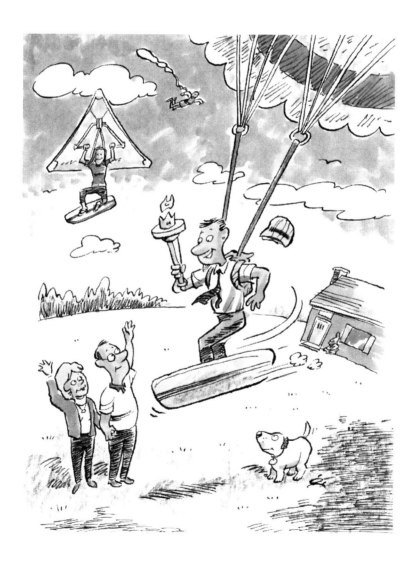

CHAPTER 24
Return of the Refugees

If all goes well, the ability to compromise and set limits will be learned and any serious accidents will be avoided. Moral, religious, and personal values will be further fine-tuned. Vocational goals will also be more reachable. The practical, realistic chores of re-packing for the trip home are now added to the ability to plan for future voyages. It is with mixed emotions that the rockets are gingerly shifted into reverse gear and cautiously restarted so that the capsule will slowly decelerate and begin a gradual downward descent.

Sometimes there is more of a backfire, or even a rare kickback all the way toward early puberty. Special commands may need to be sent up from mission control, to help talk down teens who seem to be in suspended animation or floating a bit. It will also take careful positioning for those who are spinning out of control to assume the right attitude. They need to avoid any unnecessary friction as they plunge down into an air of uncertainty and fall back into a world of reality.

Most teens prefer the sunny-side-up approach. As they are about to descend from outer space they may climb up to the observation deck for one last glimpse or close-up view of the heavens above. It's a surreal and eerie scene as they look up at the stars against a backdrop of total darkness while they are basking in the sunshine during the bright of day. There is also a feeling of serenity and peace as they listen to the sounds of silence. Even as they begin to pick up speed, a sense of stillness remains because there is no wind, no air, or no breeze to offer any resistance.

As they continue to dive back to earth, the astronauts recognize that their future is beginning to take shape and they hope that everything will fall into place. They have a spectacular, wide view of the whole planet, which may still be clouded as they stare down at the world below. As time flies by they can fall back on their support systems and personal strengths to help bring everything into better focus, and to get their bearings. This gives teens a sense of direction and feeling of stability as they stand up to the mounting pressures and rising forces during the final stages of the process of becoming mature adults.

As they come down out of thin air, adolescents will drop into a more demanding atmosphere. They will need to learn how to carry their own weight and pull their share of the load. As the forces of gravity build up and they begin to take the Gs, nobody ever guaranteed that adolescents would have a smooth ride back or a safe flight home. With thermal tiles and heat shield aglow with the friction, this is no time for teens to come out of the shell. They still need to be insulated to some degree because they are about to enter life in the cold, cruel outside world. Enough time in the incubator of the space capsule is necessary to make sure that emergence as an adult turns into everything it is cracked up to be. After all, no one wants to be stuck with a bad egg.

As the earth's atmosphere is reentered, it is time for teens to see the light. There is also a sense of fulfillment, and an appreciation for the changes that have taken place. For some teens the journey through adolescence will have been 'not too long,' while for others it will have been 'not too short.' Almost all will have precious memories to treasure or to share, when it's their turn at show and tell.

CHAPTER 25
Ready or Not, Here I Come

Home is so close, and yet so far. The reentry process can be very unsteady and even dangerous for teens who are poorly equipped or ill-prepared. As parents look up to catch a glimpse of the falling spacecraft, they must dig down deep to bury their worries and hide their worst fears. As hard as it may seem during this important time, sometimes it is better if parents just simply close their eyes or look the other way. Some may be in denial and pretend not to see. After all, handing over the controls to a bunch of beginners can be risky business, and very painful to watch. It doesn't create much confidence either, when the novice crew is playing flashlight tag, enjoying a game of hide and seek, or joining in some other merriment of youth. Adding to their parents' anxiety, many teens also seem to be hard of hearing during their last fling, and shouting into their headphones may only fall on deaf ears.

TEEN TIP – Late adolescence is a bit of an awkward stage, when you would like to be completely independent and have a place of your own but still don't quite have the money or means to do it. This is when a little extra patience brings a big reward. Don't feel pressured into making living arrangements, career commitments, or other decisions that you are not quite ready for. Enjoy the fading moments of your childhood while you can. You'll be out on your own soon enough. Even when you do grow up, you can always still be a kid at heart.

As they take charge of their life, it must be realized that adolescents should be allowed to blaze their own trail and land at their own pace. Sometimes it may seem as if teens are suffering from a hangover during this process. As the shuttle glides toward the runway they may want to circle overhead for a while and postpone the final approach to adulthood. A low cloud cover may hide the craft, but as it breaks the sound barrier a loud sonic boom will announce the grand entrance for all to hear. At first sighting, it may look like a UFO that is hovering as if to survey the terrain, or hesitating as if to pick the right spot to land on unfamiliar soil.

When they are about to leave their childhood, some teenagers will strap on a parachute and enjoy a free fall for as long as they can until they finally have to pull the ripcord. Others may frolic in the winds as they sky-surf all the way home. Still others may hitch a ride on a hang glider, hoping to catch any updrafts or rising currents as they try to defy the laws of gravity. Who can blame them? Growing up is hard to do - and the longer you can put it off, the better. This is where well timed support from the control tower comes in handy. It's quite amazing how a few encouraging words can be so useful in helping the astronauts make a gentle descent and smooth landing as their maturing process is almost complete.

PARENT TIP - The basic principles for success at this stage continue to be simple, safe, and down-to-earth. Adolescents still need you to stay connected, to show unconditional love at all times, and to have faith that they will make it back, even if left to their own devices. Don't give up now. If you can hang in there just a little bit longer, all those years of effort should finally begin to pay off.

Quarantined by the jitter bug

Beth was an 18-year-old girl I saw at the request of her pediatrician, for a 2-year history of nausea and vomiting. She was described as a very high strung and emotional young woman.

Both Beth and her mother told me that the symptoms usually occurred whenever she was tense or upset. Beth said that she felt stressed out all the time, and she would become very anxious whenever she was left alone. She also was afraid to leave the house or to have any social contacts on the outside. She would especially worry at night, and was unable to sleep alone. It was very obvious that Beth was suffering from an anxiety disorder, and that she was becoming more and more withdrawn. She was quickly becoming emotionally crippled, to the point of being homebound. She certainly was not ready to finish separating from her parents, and go out on her own.

Beth lived more than an hour away from my office, and it was hard for her to travel back and forth during the snowy winter months. She was able to connect with a therapist in her hometown who taught her various relaxation and behavior modification techniques. We worked as a team, and I prescribed medication to lessen Beth's anxiety. She checked in with me frequently, and I was able to follow much of her progress over the phone. When she came back to my office one month later she seemed to be much more outgoing and animated. It was almost like talking with a different girl.

Over a period of months Beth made dramatic improvement. She was starting to take short trips outside of the home all by herself, and was gradually increasing the time spent away from her family. She also started babysitting younger children and earning extra money. This helped her feel more independent and self-reliant. Once she learned how to drive a car life was really sweet for Beth. She certainly deserved it, after suffering for so long. Her case points out how anxiety about separating from their childhood home can be very extreme for some teens, and can even completely paralyze those who are more severely afflicted. This is particularly true in sensitive individuals like Beth, who are not ready to assume the role of an adult and need more time to finish the work of adolescence.

CHAPTER 26
Suffering from Senioritis

Education is still in the picture for many older adolescents. Teens in their last year of high school frequently come down with a case of 'Senioritis' when they start to feel the pressures of leaving the nest. They often want to slack off and have a good time as they begin to realize that this could be their last little fling with many of their friends. They sometimes feel like they are under the gun, as over-enthusiastic parents set their sights on high goals or unrealistic grades in preparation for college. These seniors may have a fear of failure and be afraid they will not be able to take care of themselves. They may even feel like they're being pushed out while they're still wet behind the ears. Nevertheless, they continue to worry about the health of family members and friends, especially since they're about to move out, go off to college, or head off for parts unknown. In fact, they often suffer from strong feelings of guilt, or mixed feelings about leaving, if any loved ones are seriously ill, handicapped, involved in an abusive relationship, etc. It is often said that three of the most traumatic events in life are death, divorce, or moving. Any combination of these factors can create a difficult problem for most teens, who do not want to abandon the family under such circumstances. They may hang around, avoid school, or put their own life on hold for a while until they are completely sure that their presence is no longer necessary.

TEEN TIP – Separating from your home and family does not follow any fixed time schedule. Whether you head out a little sooner or a little later than expected doesn't really matter in the big picture. What does matter is that your sense of purpose is fulfilled, and that you are at peace with yourself. The decision to move on or stick around to help your family is a very personal one. Trust your instincts and follow your heart so you will not have any regrets further down the line.

A belly of nerves

Bruce was an 18-year-old high school senior with a history of exhaustion and a 25-pound weight loss over a several month period. He was often nauseated, had lost his appetite, and had no energy. He was put through extensive medical tests and no underlying physical problem was found. But it became obvious that Bruce had been under plenty of stress. He said that he was working 20 hours a week at a part time job and would sometimes simply 'forget' to eat. His mother was very worried about him and her constant reminders about food created tension between the two of them. Bruce told us that he was often emotionally abused by his girlfriend, who was always putting him down. He was very sensitive and took this very much to heart. He also had frequent arguments with his father, who told him that it was time for him to go out on his own and threatened to kick him out of the house after he finished high school later that year. In addition, he was trying hard to get good enough grades so that after graduation he would have a chance of getting into college.

Bruce sensed that he was at a turning point. As he became more anxious about the future he couldn't sleep, which only added to his suffering. A state of panic began to set in and he struggled to function as he became paralyzed by his own fears. He was a very shy, quiet kid who would cry to himself rather than burden others with his problems. He was very definitely in the reentry phase of his space flight, and was beginning to feel the Gs and take the heat as part of the process of maturing. He was obviously becoming emotionally exhausted from the stress, and headed for a premature burnout. Bruce was suffering from severe anxiety, which seems to strike such kind, caring, and conscientious kids who feel as if they are carrying the weight of the world on their shoulders. It seems as if they are expected to turn into instant adults as soon as they graduate from high school or reach a certain age.

Although Bruce kept his thoughts to himself, in a sense he was screaming to be heard. Once he and I got to know each other and started communicating, he was very open and willing to talk about his feelings. With counseling Bruce and his family were able to understand that growing up is more of a gradual process that doesn't automatically happen overnight, or as soon as someone is handed a diploma. In our safe, non-judgmental office surroundings, Bruce and his parents were able to air out their differences and come to a meeting of the minds. This took a lot of the pressure off so that Bruce was actually able to enjoy his last few months of high school. It was great to see him be able to take a deep breath and let out a sigh of relief.

★★★★★★

Been there, done that! Words of encouragement from the voice of experience can be very comforting to less seasoned parents, who may be having difficulty completing the separation process. This is especially true for parents who may be suffering from any combination of sorrow, sadness, or separation anxiety of their own. As the parting moment finally arrives, they may begin a cram course when it is suddenly realized that they have not taught their son or daughter everything there is to know about going out on their own.

PARENT TIP – It's always a turning point when teens leave home for the first time. As a parent you may try to squeeze last minute advice, detailed directions, or words of wisdom into every available second. This natural and very common sense of urgency, immediacy, or panic usually serves no useful purpose and only adds to everyone's tension. This is when you need to step back, take a deep breath, and try to savor the moment. Teaching your kids what you feel they should know is a continuing process, which takes place over a lifetime. So relax – there is no deadline.

For those who go to college, it is always a dramatic scene when the new freshmen are dropped off at school and there is not a dry eye in sight. I clearly remember the words of the university president at freshman orientation when our oldest son started college. From his lofty podium the president proudly stated that college life changes a person forever. He said, "When your son or daughter comes back home he or she will be different." My wife and I looked at each other and cringed. We thought, What are you going to do to our little boy? We were not comforted by the president's scholarly advice. His choice of words offered no relief for parents who were already suffering from high anxiety. But the president turned out to be right. When our boy came back home he *had* changed – he was a man.

I also remember when my wife and I said goodbye to our youngest daughter at the airport, after she had a short winter break from school. She was upset about going back to the small community college she was attending, in a tourist town that closed down during the off-season. To make the time go faster and earn extra money, she had found a part time job at a veterinary hospital, but it was still a very cold and lonely town to live in that time of year. We tried to soothe her by saying it would not be too long before we see you again. With tears pouring down her cheeks, she said, "It won't be too short, either."

Once she got back to her apartment she felt much better because she was embraced by her fiancé, who also was very homesick. She was also greeted by five cats she had rescued while working at the vet's. They were wonderful companions, and helped get her through the rest of the academic year. Once classes were over, she stuck around; the town was bustling with tourists again and she had a chance to earn a little extra money. It was quite obvious that she had grown from the experience, and was beginning to find herself. When she did come home later in the summer, we agreed to let her bring the five cats and a puppy she had recently acquired, until she could find a place for them. Things got a little crowded; we had four cats and a dog of our own. Parents must keep telling themselves that teens do come back. But when they do, they may not be alone.

CHAPTER 27
Keeping Their Guard Up

Abuse is still a serious topic, even for older adolescents or fully grown adults. The reentry phase is no time for a letdown. There may be stowaway emotions on board, which can steal the personalities and sense of self of unsuspecting victims. While they may be out of sight, unresolved conflicts stemming from past abuse are by no means out of mind. Memories which have been buried or repressed may rise to the surface at any time, for little or no obvious reason. This is a lot of baggage and a heavy burden for anyone to carry, especially if it is hidden from others or not even obvious to the adolescents themselves. Unfortunately, the longer these deep-seated feelings stay, the harder it may be to dump them. They can be a real drag and pull teens down at a time when they are trying so hard to grow up. Such powerful feelings are often camouflaged or otherwise hidden. It may take keen instincts to smell trouble in teens who are suffering on the inside while they appear to be so happy and healthy on the outside.

The words "Seek and ye shall find" still apply to screening for abuse during the reentry period. This can be shown by a study we did on incoming first-year students at a nearby university, who were taking a pre-participation sports physical exam. Although the athletes completed the questionnaire during a fairly impersonal multi-station mass screening exam conducted by persons whom they had never met, nearly one third still admitted that they had been abused or mistreated in some way in the past. In addition, 12% of the female students disclosed that they had been sexually abused. These problems would not have been discovered using the standard forms and criteria which are recommended today for the sports physical, which is often the only medical exam that participating youth get. These results strengthen the importance of routinely screening for abuse all through adolescence, and make it clear that student athletes should have access to care where such important matters can be dealt with properly.

PARENT TIP - Adolescents in their late teens still deserve to have a comprehensive medical exam on a regular basis. This includes screening for abuse and other such sensitive issues. When it's time for a regular checkup, sports physical, or college entrance exam, take your teen to a health care professional who performs this type of in-depth evaluation on a routine basis.

Putting up a tough front

Stephanie was an 18-year-old girl who I was asked to see for evaluation of a 30-pound weight loss. She had managed to lose this amount over several weeks, by cutting way back on the amount of food she ate. I did a thorough medical exam and could find no organic cause of the severe weight loss. Stephanie told me that she felt fat, and wanted to lose even more weight. At that point she still weighed about 125 pounds so she was not in any immediate medical danger. There was no evidence of vomiting or other purging behavior, which can cause an electrolyte imbalance in the body, with a serious loss of potassium.

My nurse practitioner and I worked closely with Stephanie for several months, but we seemed to make little progress. In fact, Stephanie was losing ground because she lost another 10 pounds and dropped down to 115 pounds. Her parents were very supportive, but they were also understandably very frustrated. They were not alone, either. I clearly remember one day when the nurse practitioner came out of the room, shaking her head in frustration after spending about an hour with Stephanie.

Stephanie's illness had taken a firm grip, and she was arguing with her parents more and more. We then asked a therapist to work with Stephanie and her family. He was able to work out a temporary cease-fire in the fighting, which seemed to give everyone a little time to catch their breath.

But after a few weeks Stephanie became more defiant, and more depressed. One night her father called me at my home and said that she had just cut her wrists. The wounds were very shallow and he was sure that they did not need stitches. I then spoke with Stephanie and her mother. After a rather long talk we all decided that she would be safe at home that night, as long as her parents took turns watching her. They felt comfortable that they could physically protect her if she tried to hurt herself again. They also knew that they could call the police or an ambulance to take her to our hospital for emergency psychiatric care before the situation got out of control at home. Fortunately, nothing else happened that night.

I saw Stephanie the next morning and she seemed much better. She had stayed up most of the night talking to her parents. She was very relieved that she was able to open up to them, and that they were willing to listen to her. We set up a meeting with the family therapist. I attended the session along with Stephanie, her parents, and her brother. We were able to buy a little time, since Stephanie was no longer actively suicidal.

The therapist and I kept close watch on Stephanie for several weeks. We met with her and the family several times, trying to get more understanding into what was bothering her. Something seemed to be missing, but we just couldn't put our finger on it.

Stephanie continued to struggle. The therapist, my nurse practitioner, and I finally decided to admit to her a psychiatric hospital for more intensive treatment. She spent 10 weeks in this facility, and the bill came to $85,000. She wasn't cured, but her eating disorder was much better and she was medically stable.

Her parents then asked me about sending Stephanie to a therapist who could see her one-on-one, because they felt that they couldn't do any more good working together with the family therapist. This seemed reasonable to me, and the right arrangements were made. Stephanie and her parents hit it off very well with the new therapist, but after several sessions he did not have good news for them. He diagnosed Stephanie as having a borderline personality and conduct disorder. He stated that the treatment would take a long time, and that there was no guarantee it would cure her. He gave the parents different suggestions on setting limits, and how to deal with any manipulative behaviors. Needless to say they were not thrilled with the therapist's diagnosis, although they accepted it.

I lost track of Stephanie when the medical concerns were resolved, and she returned to the care of her family physician. Several years passed, and I ran into her father by chance. He said that his daughter was finally doing much better. She had eventually been able to admit to her parents that she had been raped by a neighborhood boy shortly before all of her symptoms started. She had been unable to tell anyone about this previously. I wondered why she didn't confide in me, since we had a good relationship and I had asked her directly about any history of abuse. The father told me that she couldn't have told me even if she wanted to. He said she had been so emotionally damaged by the rape that the memories had been completely buried. He then thanked me for sticking by her and helping the family get through the most difficult times.

At last the missing piece to the puzzle had been found. Symptoms of sexual abuse and other such emotionally damaging events can closely imitate certain features of a borderline personality disorder. It is not known how often this occurs, but the number of times has probably been greatly underestimated. Emotional abuse can be just as stressful as physical abuse for children and adolescents. It's really not too surprising that youth who have been subjected to such traumatic events may put up such a tough exterior, or seem to have a bit of an attitude. On the inside they are very sensitive people with deep emotional wounds which need to be healed. These teens are often on the defensive, and often overreact to things so that they will not get hurt even more.

Once Stephanie was able to work through the issues around the rape she began to improve dramatically. She started to act like her old self, and was much more sociable once again. She graduated from college and found a good job, which involved working closely with the public. She was psychologically and socially intact - so much for the incorrect diagnosis of borderline personality disorder. It was time throw away the label, and for Stephanie to get on with her life.

161

★★★★★★

Date rape is now the most common form of rape for adolescents. More than half of those seen in rape crisis centers report that the assault occurred on a date - in most instances, the first date. The victims usually know the attacker, feel coerced into having sex, and feel partially responsible for the situation. It has been shown that the risk of rape is greater if the male asks the female out, pays for the date, and drives the car. As with younger adolescents, there is often a strong relationship between sexual assault and the use of alcohol or other drugs by the victims themselves, as well as by their assailants. The latest forget-me pills or similar drugs, new weapons to dope young women and make them defenseless, have taken date rape to an even sleazier level. Of course the same concerns also apply to gay and bisexual youth.

TEEN TIP – Don't be an easy target. The facts speak for themselves. If you are drunk or out of it, you become the perfect prey. Rapists and other perpetrators thrive on victims who are not in their right senses. Even well meaning individuals can get carried away under such circumstances. To reduce your risks, you need to be in control. Staying away from drugs and keeping sober are still your best defense.

CHAPTER 28
Wanted: Sober Genes

D rugs and other decoys often clutter the astronauts' return path to life in the real world. The ability to resist such temptations is often handed down from one generation to the next. As adolescent substance abusers come down from their orbit above, it must be remembered that problems with alcohol and other drugs only start up at this age. The use of alcohol, marijuana, cocaine, and other illegal chemicals occurs in all levels of our society, which makes a heavy burden for the young, the restless, and the impressionable. They are destined to crash land unless we as a society are able to lighten their load by reducing their need for instant gratification, and for feeling perfect all the time. After all, maybe there is something to be said for having a bad hair day every now and then. It is time to dissolve the myths, defend the susceptible targets and decontaminate the victims of this worldwide assault. This is a form of chemical warfare. It will be won in the mind, not on the street!

TEEN TIP – Studies show that alcoholism runs in families-- alcoholics are much more likely than nonalcoholics to have blood relatives who are alcohol dependent. This genetic inclination to alcoholism can be very powerful and sometimes even all consuming. This is a fact, not an excuse to follow in the footsteps of family members who have already taken the bait and fallen into the trap. As you become your own person, in the end you will need to answer only to yourself. Consuming alcohol is not a healthy response to peer pressure or a good solution to your personal problems. Once the habit of drinking takes hold, a life of deceit and denial are likely to follow. The bottle becomes your master and there is no longer a sense of responsibility to anyone, including yourself. To stay in control of your life, keep a clear head and think, don't drink.

Drowning in a pool of tears

Kevin was an 18-year-old boy whose pediatrician sent him to me because he had pain in his abdomen, nausea, diarrhea, headaches, dizziness, and anxiety. I did an in-depth medical history, psychosocial profile, and physical exam. Kevin had just been seen by a specialist of the stomach and intestines, who put him on medication for what he believed was stress-related intestinal problems. This treatment worked very quickly, and Kevin got a lot of relief from the pain, nausea, and diarrhea. But after a complete evaluation it soon became obvious that his other symptoms were related to stress and anxiety as well. Kevin also openly admitted that he was very tense, and felt like he was under a lot of pressure.

Kevin and I then talked about the underlying issues in greater detail. He had been diagnosed as having attention deficit hyperactivity disorder (ADHD), and was doing very poorly in school. He had been put on medication for this, but there had been no real improvement. He was a very intelligent, deep thinking young man who felt out of place in the classroom. He loved walking in the woods and being close to nature. The thought of going to school often made him so nervous that he would feel too sick to go. As the absences began to pile up he felt even more overwhelmed, and he finally dropped out of school.

Kevin was very creative and would spend day after day expressing his feelings through his drawings. He told me that he did his best work when he was angry and upset. He had a short temper and was easily irritated by others. He got into several fights when he was in school and boasted that he always came out on top. Kevin was a tall, wiry kid, and his mother told me, "Nobody messes with him." He was an enthusiastic hunter with an unusual appreciation for nature. He had ready access to guns, knives, and other weapons, which was a reason to be concerned because of his inner anger. He took after his grandfather, who was a great outdoorsman and who taught him everything he knew about the wild. The two were very close and would spend a lot of time hunting together. Tragically, his grandfather had been found dead in the woods several years before. Kevin had never been the same since, according to his mother.

As I got to know Kevin a little better it became clear that he was not only suffering from stress and anxiety, but from depression and despair as well. He had unresolved grief over the loss of his grandfather and felt there was no one to turn to for help. The depth of his sorrow had gone unrecognized for many years. I did not really know how bad he was hurting until one day when Kevin was leaning on a small table in the exam room with his face buried under his arms as we talked. As he raised his head I noticed a small drop of moisture on the table. Before I knew it there was a pool of tears. Kevin then began to sob as he described how sad he had been for so many years. I explained to him that I was able to feel his pain and that we could work through his troubles with the help of a therapist. He was not suicidal, so there was some time to work out the issues.

Kevin had a lot going on in his head. His parents had been divorced for several years and he was living with his mother. He would frequently get into arguments with her about common, everyday things like cleaning his room and picking up after himself. The fact that Kevin quit school seemed to make both of them even more frustrated. The mother was working several jobs just to make ends meet, and she was exhausted when she got home. She could not afford to buy him all the clothes he wanted and Kevin was only able to find odd jobs to earn money every now and then. They loved one another very much, but the strain was starting to show and beginning to take a toll on both of them.

Kevin was also a bit of a pothead. He smoked marijuana every day, trying to calm down. He also got drunk fairly often, to try and forget about his problems. Basically, he was doing what is called 'self-medicating.' He saw his father on a regular basis, but he was not able to talk openly with him or feel that he had a shoulder to lean on. Kevin's dad believed that most of his son's troubles were caused by the marijuana, instead of the other way around. He felt that Kevin would do much better if he could learn how to relax and calm down without getting high. The father was also worried that Kevin had inherited the tendency to heavy drinking and chemical dependency, because his older brother's use of drugs and alcohol was out of control.

Kevin and his parents made a good connection with the family therapist. They were able to work through the issues that were adding to his stress, anxiety, and depression. We also used medication for these symptoms, because Kevin was suffering so badly that he was barely able to function.

After a few months he felt much better, and the situation at home had improved greatly. Kevin's keen sense of humor, which had been gone for so long, came back. As he continued to get better the medication was stopped, and the visits to the therapist were spaced out. The last time I heard from Kevin he was holding his own and working on getting his diploma so he could go to college. He also no longer used alcohol or marijuana to change his mood. Gene therapy aside, this case shows how a dose of happiness can be an extremely effective weapon for lowering the risk of chemical dependency.

PARENT TIP – Set a good example for your kids. It's not good enough to speak out against alcohol and other drugs. You need to show them by your actions. If you must drink, then do so in moderation and make every effort to safeguard your supply of alcohol from curious teens. If you drink and drive while under the influence, don't be surprised if your adolescents do the same thing. Likewise, if you hop into the passenger seat when the driver is drunk or high, you are sending a dangerous message. While you may not always be able to stop your teenager from drinking, you don't need to encourage or approve of this behavior either. It's up to you to set the rules, and lay down the law when the rules are broken.

CHAPTER 29
Designated Drivers or Designated Dupes?

Safety practices do not always follow the ground rules. The reentry process is much more difficult for the group of older teens who are in the habit of getting soused or smashed. Their landing gear may not be completely open and their thought patterns may be somewhat disturbed or relatively strung out, even when they are sober. Adolescents frequently have a twisted, mistaken view of alcohol-related driving risk, and often underestimate the negative influence of alcohol use on driving. Many believe that alcohol will not have any effect on driving behavior, and some even feel that alcohol will actually improve their driving. In a survey that we conducted on 138 first year student athletes at a university in upstate New York, a quarter of them said that they had driven a motor vehicle after drinking or using drugs. In addition, over 40% of the students had been a passenger when the driver was drunk or high. Drugs, drinking, and driving are never a good mix, especially for teens who are looking for direction as they head into a topsy-turvy world. They need to hang tough, gain a wide view of life, and search for the truth with a clear head and an open mind. Otherwise they may fall into a trap, suffer from tunnel vision, and develop a narrow outlook with a twisted view of reality. They may create quite a stir as they go into a tailspin, get turned upside down or come in for a belly landing. Sometimes they wind up dead on arrival. It's hard to get the whole picture or stay in one piece when the pilot is plastered.

Teens need to develop a survival plan to avoid harm. In the short run, the use of designated drivers is a very attractive idea that has saved many lives. Over the long haul, though, it has probably ruined many more by giving teens the idea that it is okay to get drunk, even if you are underage, as long as you don't drive. This is the wrong message for adolescents. Although designated drivers may have the best intentions, they are basically enablers for problem drinkers who may go on to a lifelong habit of alcoholism or addiction. The designated driver idea should not be completely thrown out; it's an important emergency plan for isolated, unexpected times when there aren't any other choices. In a pinch, I would certainly advise teens to use this method. But designated drivers should not be used as the *main* plan in the fight against DWI - it's winning the battle, but losing the war.

TEEN TIP - Be a survivor. Have your safety plan in place before you go out with your friends. While the use of designated drivers may seem like a good idea, staying sober should always be the top plan. Never get behind the wheel after using alcohol or other drugs, and don't get into the car when the driver is under the influence. As a backup, be sure you have someone to call at any hour of the day or night if you need a ride home. Carry a cell phone or enough change to make the call, when necessary. Whatever you do, don't walk home on unsafe roads, especially at night. Bring warm clothes along in cold weather in case you need to wait outdoors for your ride.

It's time to get strict in other areas too. Colleges that let booze flow in dorms, fraternities, and university functions are really only looking to fill in their own bottom line and make a profit. By looking the other way and ignoring the drinking, they are certainly not thinking about the health or wellbeing of their students. The term 'dry campus' seems to be a dirty word among colleges, especially when it comes to looking for new students. Colleges need tuition to survive, and because of the heavy competition for students, many schools seem to be afraid that if they don't allow drinking, young people will go instead to colleges that do allow it. It's no wonder there are so many party animals running around in student bodies these days. In the war on drugs, these schools have decided to take a self-defensive position, and allow their use. Its time to stop this foxhole mentality by rewarding money to universities that are willing to take a stand and make a preventative strike against substance abuse on the front lines. The powerful brain trusts of institutions of higher learning need to get back to the drawing board if the standards of their university are being lowered to those of just another party school. With a little creativity and a lot of commitment they should be able to capture the attention of bright, fun loving students who have their priorities straight. After all, nobody wants to be stuck with a bunch of deadbeats or party poopers.

Surviving by default

Anthony was an 18-year-old boy who came in to my office for a routine physical exam. He seemed very anxious when I shook hands with him and introduced myself. His mother told me that he didn't have any medical problems, but she was very concerned about his lack of direction, his impatience, and the fact that he had trouble controlling his anger. She was raising him with the help of her sister, because his father wasn't around any more. There was a lot of stress and tension in the home, so this was getting harder. Also, for a long time Anthony had had trouble learning, and had been recently diagnosed with attention deficit hyperactivity disorder (ADHD). It was getting harder and harder for him to pay attention to his schoolwork. He couldn't keep up with the other students at school, and his grades were poor.

Anthony's exam showed that physically he was completely normal, but it was soon obvious that he had problems. He and his mother would often get into loud arguments. When he told me how she did not give him much freedom, he got very emotional and started to pound his fist into his hand. At home things would quickly get out of hand whenever he stayed out later than his curfew. He and his mother would scream and swear at each another. Anthony was a big, strong young man and his mother was afraid for her safety during his fits of anger. He never hurt her, but her worry made sense because his temper tantrums were happening more often, and getting worse.

But underneath this tough front was a tender teen with very low self-esteem. Anthony's athletic abilities made him feel good about himself, and he had experimented with anabolic steroids to improve his performance. He dreamed of going to college on a baseball scholarship. He was an excellent pitcher, but he had recently injured his throwing arm and could no longer compete at his usual performance level. He seemed quite upset and bitter about this bad luck. He now felt that he had no future in sports, and he wasn't sure that he would get good enough grades to graduate that year. In an act of despair, Anthony gave up and dropped out of school.

Anthony then turned to alcohol and marijuana as a source of comfort. He would often get drunk or high with his friends and would frequently get into fights. He got into trouble with the law when he beat up another youth during a drunken brawl. He was arrested and charged with assault. But this did not seem to slow him down, and he kept drinking heavily. Fortunately, he had enough sense to not get behind the wheel, or ride as a passenger when the driver was under the influence. He would often call his mother and ask her to give him a ride home. He knew he could count on her to be a default driver in these situations.

His mother, though, had been pushed to the limit with these late night escapades. She refused to bail him out any more, because she believed that by driving him home she was helping him to keep drinking and, in effect, becoming an enabler. To some extent this was true, but more importantly she was also a lifesaver for her son.

I encouraged the mother to continue to respond to her son's calls for help in such situations. These were not times to confront him or to pass judgement. The object was to get him home safely and let him sleep it off. I explained that we could sit down and work out the different problems when everyone had cooled down. This is all part of the survival plan.

The mother got the message and realized that failure to answer her son's SOS signals could result in serious injury or even death. I found a family therapist to help sort out the underlying issues and cool off the crisis atmosphere in the home. I also met alone with Anthony to try to improve his self-esteem, so he would feel less need to get a boost from alcohol or other drugs. The last time I saw him, the plan seemed to be working and things at home had become fairly calm.

★★★★★★

Every effort must be made to prevent the problem behavior described in Anthony's case, but other backup plans must be ready in case the usual efforts don't work. This is where the idea of having an emergency, default driver ready, even late at night, makes sense. While the prevention of driving under the influence must always be the most important goal, the default driver does a necessary, lifesaving job by providing a safe ride home before anyone gets too far bent out of shape. Designated drivers can actually encourage drinking because they go along for the night out so others can drink. But a default driver does not go along, and is to be called only when there is a need. Default drivers do not really encourage drinking because they do not promote chemical dependency up front, and only help teens who need a ride after their use of alcohol or other drugs has already occurred.

PARENT TIP – Remember, educating your kids is a continual process. Don't allow underage drinking in your home, and always discourage adolescents from attending any activities where this is likely to occur. Keep reminding them of the dangers of drinking and drugs, especially when operating a motor vehicle. Reinforce the importance of staying straight and keeping sober as the top survival strategy. Be sure they have a backup plan in place, just in case this first layer of protection breaks down. This would include having someone to call for a safe ride home so that they will not be forced into a dangerous situation when the driver's judgement is impaired.

CHAPTER 30
Hello, Good Buddy

riends gradually drop out of the scene during this stage, since security in numbers is no longer needed. As adolescence winds down, the young adventurers begin to pair up as the search for a soul mate becomes more intense. A few couples are ready for a permanent commitment at this point, but most are not quite ready to completely settle down. It is common for them to play the field and jump from one partner to another because they are still a little flighty at this stage. Peer pressure becomes less important, and adolescents become more choosy about their companions. They may hang out with a few old pals or develop a few new friendships.

While teens are developing minds of their own, they may start to stumble or wonder exactly where they stand. As parents come back into the picture, there is generally re-acceptance of their advice and greater appreciation of their experience. Small amounts of encouragement and reassurance from parents can give a big lift to youths with deflated egos. With their newly found intelligence and wisdom, parents are now better able to help guide their teens down the final pathway to self-discovery.

TEEN TIP – It's quite natural to have a bit of an empty feeling as you and your friends head out in different directions. The less time you have to sit and think about it, the better. This is when you need to stay busy by getting a job, furthering your education, or getting involved in other similar activities to occupy your time. If you need a little break before you start, then go ahead and take some time off, but set a target date so that any future plans are not put on permanent hold. Remember, you are about to become an adult so you need to begin to think like one. Don't worry if you are not ready to focus on a particular career at this point. Keep all your choices open and buy a little time until everything starts to fall into place.

Growing apart

Roxanne was an 18-year-old girl referred to me by her pediatrician, for treatment of an eating disorder. She had lost over 40 pounds in the previous six months by cutting way back on her food. She did this because she felt fat all over, especially in the lower belly.

She told me that she was not vomiting or purging in other ways and she was not using any diet pills. While she did not feel that there was any trigger factor or event, like abuse, it was obvious that this was a highly emotional time for Roxanne. She felt pressured by her parents to leave home and go off to college. Unfortunately, she wasn't ready and didn't know how to tell them.

Roxanne felt very different from other girls, and was especially upset that her closest friends were starting to drink a lot. Once a close knit group, they seemed to be growing apart and going their separate ways. The strong peer support that she had enjoyed in the past was now missing. She felt that her friends were no longer there for her and that she had no one in whom she could confide.

When I first met her, Roxanne was extremely anxious and apprehensive. In fact, she was one of the most anxious adolescents I had ever seen. She was sitting on the edge of her seat and was so nervous that she could barely speak.

Physically, Roxanne was in much better shape. Other than being nervous, her exam showed that there was nothing wrong physically. Her weight was 130 pounds, and she was in no immediate medical danger.

After the physical she seemed more relaxed, and we were able to carry on a healthy conversation. She was able to talk about how upset she had been and how hard it was to keep everything inside. She was having trouble sleeping and was beginning to feel drained. She was also getting more depressed, although she had no thoughts of suicide. I told Roxanne that I could feel her pain and that I would do everything I could to help her get through this difficult time in her life.

I saw Roxanne for several visits. I kept close watch for any physical complications and could not find any evidence of a hidden medical condition. Her weight also remained stable.

As we got better acquainted it was obvious that she was very grateful for the extra support. She was also being seen by a therapist, and a psychiatrist who was prescribing her medication. She had been on several different pills for the anxiety and depression before the right combination was found for her.

With intensive outpatient treatment, the use of modern drug therapy, and the ability to buy a little time until the medication took effect, Roxanne gradually began to feel better. Although she was not exactly excited about the possibility, she was able to attend a community college that fall. This was a big step for a young woman who was once on her last legs and headed for a breakdown.

PARENT TIP – The presence of parents as a steadying force helps to fill the void as older teenagers and their friends start to go their separate ways. Your adolescents need to know that you are still there for them to fall back on, if necessary. It's best if you let them approach you at their own pace, rather than for you to put too much pressure on them at this point. You need to listen to what they have to say, and remember that their plans for the future may not always be the same as your dreams for them. Some kids are not quite ready to automatically leave home once they reach a certain age. If you had your heart set on your adolescent going away to college after graduating from high school, get over it. Community colleges or other local schools are excellent alternatives for those who wish to further their education, but prefer to do so closer to home. If their grades are okay, they can always transfer to an out-of-town institution at a later date, if they want to.

CHAPTER 31
Finding Themselves

Image is still important during the reentry phase, but it is no longer as important as it once was. Older adolescents are less preoccupied with their personal appearance as they are about to reach adulthood and they begin to recognize who they really are. There is now a greater acceptance of the pubertal changes that have taken place, and a growing need to become a unique individual. Most of the returning astronauts have learned how to roll with the punches, duck away from improper comments, and shrug their shoulders at nasty remarks. As they start to gear down, there is also a sense of pride and anticipation because they will soon be able to go out on their own. During final preparations for landing, many are eager to have a new look to polish their image. What's different now is that slight changes in the way things are will carry them a long way. Some girls may even want their hips back. Some boys are willing to let go of the need to have a perfectly defined muscular body. Others may begin to behave like a chip off the old block, and actually imitate the parents they had ignored or even avoided during their space flight. Those who have not yet reclaimed the controls from eating disorders, body image concerns, or other issues of self-esteem may need to get ready to bail out of the capsule, or be diverted for an emergency landing. Sometimes these adolescents require complicated repairs or even a complete overhaul before they can complete the mission successfully and arrive safely at the home base.

Sorrow beyond a heartbeat

Hal was an 18-year-old whose doctor sent him to one of our heart specialists because the boy had a low heart rate. Hal was a very competitive swimmer and had no trouble keeping up with his teammates. His heart was found to be completely normal, and the cardiologist felt that his slow heart rate was a natural physical response to the fact that Hal had recently lost 20 pounds over a fairly short period of time. The cardiologist sent him to me because he was worried that Hal was quite thin and might have an eating disorder.

On my exam he did look skinny, but he was not really wasted. He seemed to be a little anxious. His face was pale, his hands were cold, and his body temperature was extremely low. As I listened to his heart, it seemed like forever between each beat: Hal's heart rate was only 35, which was the lowest rate I had ever seen in a patient who was having no symptoms of a heart problem. His body was in an energy-saving condition, with hypothermia and a slow pulse slowing down the needs of his metabolism, because of the weight loss. The rest of his physical exam was entirely normal, and all lab tests were negative.

But Hal's emotional state was another matter. He had been under an awful lot stress at home. His parents had just separated, and the family was in complete confusion. His mother had left his father for another woman. After nearly 20 years of marriage she had discovered that she was a lesbian. The situation was extremely stressful for all of the family members, especially Hal. He was a very sensitive young man who could not understand why this was happening. He was too upset to eat or sleep. He was very sad and unhappy. As is so often is the case, he wondered what he had done to cause this difficult situation. The answer was nothing! It was not his fault, although he felt somehow to blame.

I got Hal and his family into therapy right away. They were all very open and frank. The parents were able to explain to their children how they felt, and why they felt that way. Hal had taken his parents' struggle on as his own, and held it inside himself so much that his stomach was a ball of nerves, which seemed to be tied in knots. It's no wonder he wasn't able to take in enough food.

As the issues were talked out in therapy Hal gradually began to feel better, eat more, and slowly regain the weight he had lost. Once he had 'more fuel in the furnace' his heart rate went up to his regular baseline of 56, and his body temperature became normal. He graduated from high school and went off to college, and the last I heard, had become quite muscular. Better yet, he was very happy.

PARENT TIP - Never underestimate how much your kids care about you. They may not always be able to say it directly, but they do care. When you struggle, so do they. This is especially true for sensitive teenagers who tend to take on other's problems and internalize them as their own. Stay alert, since this is one of the causes for an eating disorder during adolescence. The solution is to deal with the underlying issues rather than simply focusing on any obvious eating worries.

Honoring a commitment

Katie was an 18-year-old nursing student who was dealing with an enormous amount of stress. Her mother was suffering with multiple sclerosis (MS) and her father had recently been diagnosed with a brain tumor. They were both totally disabled and becoming more dependent on her. She was trying her best to keep up her grades so that she would be able to graduate and get a job to help them out. During this struggle she developed an eating disorder with severe limiting of her food intake and vomiting of almost everything that she did eat. She lost weight at a very rapid and dangerous rate. When I first saw her she was already down to 74 pounds and she looked bad, very bad. There was no question in my mind that she was going to die if she was not hospitalized immediately.

I told Katie and her parents that she needed to be hospitalized. Her mom and dad understood the need of this decision and supported it but somehow Katie was able to convince them otherwise, and they changed their mind. This created a very difficult problem for me because I could not morally, ethically, or professionally let her go home in the condition she was in.

After discussing Katie's case with several other doctors we all realized that she needed to be committed to a psychiatric unit, with medical backup. This wasn't going to be pretty. The necessary legal papers were obtained and the police had to be called. When they showed up it was a typical busy day in the office, with many young children and adolescents around. Katie fell to the floor and began begging and pleading as she screamed to her parents, "Don't let them take me, don't let them take me!" The cops were polite, but firm. One of the officers told Katie that they had a job to do and that they could do it the easy way or the hard way. She still did not give in. Finally, when they started to haul her off, she realized they meant business and gave up, no longer fighting.

Katie spent two weeks in the psychiatric unit and was discharged too early when her insurance ran out. Arrangements were made for her to be seen by a therapist closer to her home, which was in a small town about an hour away from my office. She was still mad at me for committing her and did not want to come back to our center in Syracuse. Who could blame her? I remember thinking: This is it, she'll never make it and I'll never see her again.

I was wrong on both counts! Katie did make it. Somehow her short time in the psychiatric unit had broken the cycle, and she had gradually improved and responded to outpatient therapy. Several years passed before I heard from her again. One day she called me and said she was now a nurse working on the 8th floor of the same hospital that I was based in. She wanted me to come up and see her. I remember thinking to myself that I wasn't sure I really wanted to do this. After all, I had committed Katie to a psychiatric institution against her will and I wasn't sure why she wanted to see me again. I decided to take her up on this anyway and braced myself for the worst.

I walked up three flights of stairs to her floor. As I arrived at the nurses' station I was not really ready for what I saw; an attractive young nurse smiling from ear to ear. It was Katie. She said that she wanted to see if I would recognize her. She proudly reported that her weight was 145 pounds. I certainly didn't recognize her as she literally weighed twice as much as when I last saw her crawling on the floor and being dragged off by the cops.

Katie said she also wanted to thank me for helping her, and that she would be forever grateful. That was a big reward for walking up a few flights of stairs!

CHAPTER 32

From the Mosh Pit
to the Medic's Tent

Recreation and relaxation are food for the body and mind, and it needs to be built into the reentry phase. Before adolescents are able to settle down they often need a little more time to pause and think about things. Some may head off to the meadows to seek peace and tranquility. Others may exchange food for thought and go on a picnic or have a cookout. Throwing a tailgate party is another popular pastime, especially at rock-a-thons, where concert goers who are not quite ready to face the music can find any excuse to get tanked in the parking lot.

Others are more eager to get in the middle of things, and can't wait to beat the band. More adventurous souls will cast their fate to the wind and let themselves get carried away by the crowd. For them there's nothing like getting all lathered up on a hot summer day and body surfing to the sounds of their favorite rock bands. It's fascinating to watch them ride the tops of the waves of waving arms and hands. They look like beach balls bouncing all around as they are tossed and turned through the lively, excited crowd. The trouble is that this is strictly a spur of the moment activity, and there are no spotters or safe landing sites built into the performance. Those who are thrown up on the stage or who wind up a little short may land hard enough to see stars. When their heads clear it's time to check the body parts, pick up the pieces, and be patched up in the first aid tent if necessary.

One for the road

As an adolescent medicine specialist I've always felt that there's nothing like seeing a rock concert up close and personal. One hot day during the summer of 1998, my 14-year-old son talked my wife and I into taking him to an outdoor concert. Of course, he needed to bring a friend along. The other boy's parents believed that with the right supervision this could be a valuable educational experience. As it turned out, they were absolutely correct - my wife and I learned a lot that day. We felt very privileged since not every mom or dad has an opportunity to see such a spectacle.

As we pulled into the pasture to park the van I knew that we were all in for a real treat. It had rained heavily, and our first job was to keep from getting stuck in the mud. This was a bit tricky because there were empty beer bottles and cans scattered all over the place. There was also the odor of freshly cut hay and burning grass, with enough smoke to cloud our senses. Then there were the people - nothing but 18- to 21-year-olds running all over the place. Many were barely dressed - to beat the heat, of course. They seemed very intent on having a good time with one another and appeared totally indifferent to any grown-ups who were wandering around.

I found a fairly safe place to park and we headed off for the main gate. As we walked up to the entrance to the show we had to be checked by security - ladies first, of course. I'll never forget the look on my wife's face while she was being frisked from head to toe very thoroughly. Only a strip search would have been more complete. She was not too amused by this, but the boys and I actually thought it was pretty funny. I guess we didn't look quite as suspicious because we three guys passed through relatively untouched.

To me, the sideshows were almost as entertaining as the bands. My wife and I stood on the side so we could take it all in. The fans, the food, and the drinks by themselves didn't seem all that unusual. It was an entirely different story when they were all mixed together. There were roped off areas around the tents where alcohol was sold. Many of the booze customers looked and acted like animals in a pen. While drinking was only allowed in these special areas, it was quite obvious that there were many escapees wandering aimlessly around. As they wobbled by, they would often look at us with a blank stare. I would ask, "Hello, is anybody home?" Most usually answered with a warm, happy smile that seemed to say it all. Even as the temperature rose into the mid-90s tempers didn't rise to any degree, and everyone seemed to keep their cool.

As a doctor, I am a trained observer. My job is to study human nature. So, on that hot and humid afternoon, I did what I do best - observe. Unfortunately my wife did not always approve of what I was observing, and would move me on. She led me to a seat in the grandstand - to protect me from the sun, of course. We sat down for a few minutes and enjoyed a nice cold drink. It was very refreshing. Then we headed for the restrooms. The different sights, sounds, and chants reminded me of my college days. I got wedged into a herd of guys all crammed together in a narrow chute, trying to outmaneuver each other to reach the urinal. Some made it and some did not. As for the ladies' room, let's just say I got the better end of the deal. I guess that's why so many of the more experienced veterans simply take relief in the great outdoors at such events.

Having survived the restroom ordeal, we then headed back to listen to the bands. The volume on the jumbo speakers was set loud enough to be heard all the way to the next galaxy. I guess that's why we refer to the groups as rock stars.

The fans in the mosh pit were truly in another world. They were pressed so close together that there was barely enough room to get any air let alone take a deep breath every now and then. It's no wonder so many were waving their hands over their heads - they were probably signaling to get tossed into the air for a moment of relief.

And they did get tossed. I had never seen so many human missiles as prone, horizontal bodies were passed quickly along the top of the sea of waving hands. The close-knit members of the audience served as a giant trampoline for those who wanted another shot. They also served as a giant stretcher to pass any casualties up front, to the side of the stage. The wounded would then be tossed into the arms of the waiting medic and whisked away to a makeshift emergency shelter. All totaled there were many broken bones, cuts, and other injuries. Fortunately, most were not very serious.

Everything said and done, we all had a lot of fun. The boys really loved the music and they both took home a souvenir. I enjoyed studying all the sights and sampling the various foods. My wife had a good time too and she was especially pleased with her date.

As we made our way to the exit we were all very thirsty. The ride home would be a couple of hours, so we all bought sodas to drink in the car. As we wandered through the last security point on the way out I heard a woman say harshly, "Not so fast mister. You can't take those drinks with you." I was completely puzzled. "They might contain alcohol," she barked.

When I told her that they were just sodas she asked, "How do I know you're not lying?"

I was highly offended and gave her a piece of my mind. I was just going to dump the cup at her feet when my wife yanked me away. Cooler heads prevailed and we all reluctantly threw our drinks into the trashcan.

As we got into the van my eardrums were still vibrating from the noise and my blood was still boiling from the brush with the security woman. We were all also still very thirsty. That had to wait though, because the line of cars getting out of the pasture was extremely long. This gave me even more time to steam and fume, since it was really hot inside the car. When we rolled down the windows to cool off there was a gentle breeze carrying the aroma of manure from a nearby field. This only added to the ambience.

Then it hit me that I wasn't really mad at the security guard. The remarks she made were typical of a society that is rapidly decomposing, just like the cow pies. Seeing so many concert goers getting drunk or stoned was very troubling to me. Losing the freedom to have a soda for the road was even more disturbing since it was an insult to my integrity. Then again, a culture of chemical people doesn't carry a conscience.

This story shows how the widespread use of alcohol by adolescents is not only permitted in our society, it is actually encouraged. This is exactly the opposite message that should be given to young people today. A more aggressive, preventative approach to fighting adolescent alcohol abuse is needed to reverse today's values about alcohol. Politically, the prevention of underage drinking must be considered a top priority by local, state, and federal officials. Existing laws must be consistently enforced if they are to become more effective. Extra resources need to be given to authorities so they have more manpower to catch people involved in illegal sales or purchases. Violations must have harsher penalties, and offenders must be prosecuted to the full extent of the law. As always, a strong family is the best defense against substance abuse and other such risk-taking behaviors during adolescence. Promotion of healthy recreation habits to help relieve stress is an important part of this plan.

PARENT TIP - Although adolescents are young and energetic, they can still experience burnout at any point along the line. As they take on more responsibility, they need to have some time to relax and unwind, just like adults. For teens who are already trying their hardest, it usually does not help to keep reminding them about not 'performing up to their potential.' In fact, adolescents often shudder at the sound of these words since they are sometimes just another source of extra pressure. Be supportive and encourage them to do their best, but don't expect them to perform well if they are pushed beyond their limits.

★★★★★★

Adolescents who are living on luck may need more than a good bookie. Problem gambling has become a serious issue for young adults. Many grown-ups can't understand why adolescents leave so much to chance. Quite frankly, they have had good teachers and have learned their lessons well. Legalized gambling is an excellent example. Casinos are being built all over the country. They are open 24 hours a day, offer a glittery atmosphere, and provide great food at bargain prices. Once inside, younger customers may be especially tempted to take a spin at the wheel, roll the dice on the table, or toss a coin into the slot machine.

State lotteries are also growing by leaps and bounds. Tickets can be bought at local convenience stores, and the cost is whatever the buyer can bear. For most customers, buying an occasional lottery ticket is just innocent fun and simple entertainment. Money produced from lotteries is often used to help fund public education and other worthy causes. But those who see gambling as a way to bail their state out of a fiscal crisis are very shortsighted. From the public health point of view, long-term strategies for cutting frivolous spending, or raising taxes, are far better ways to balance the budget. While the entrepreneurs and government officials are filling their own pockets, they are actually also stealing the sense of self of adolescents who have a tendency toward compulsive gambling. What may have started out as an innocent $1 bet may wind up as a lifelong habit for those who get hooked. It may be easy for these teenagers to make a simple bet or to follow a hot tip, but it will take much more than a little luck to beat the odds and overcome their addiction.

TEEN TIP - If you obsess about money or are prone to compulsive behaviors, you are at risk for becoming a problem gambler. This can develop into a serious addiction that can use all of your energy and take control of your life. It's very easy to get started with a little bet here and there. Before you know it, you could be in over your head in debt. Remember, when you enter the world of organized gambling, the odds are always stacked in favor of the house, and against the gambler. In all probability, you will come out on the losing end.

CHAPTER 33
Sowing their Oats

S exuality issues such as unplanned pregnancies and the spread of sexually transmitted diseases(STDs) continue to be major concerns at this stage. During the reentry phase, peer group involvement becomes less important and there is a tendency to look for close, more intimate personal relationships as part of this process. Practical plans for contraception and disease prevention must remain in place for immediate use as needed. Saving sex, postponing sexual involvement, and practicing second virginity continue to be the most effective ways to meet these goals. Access to emergency birth control must also still be available for use when specifically indicated.

TEEN TIP - If you have not yet been sexually active, you have made a wise choice from the medical perspective. '*Not* doing it' is still the best thing *to* do, to eliminate the possibility of an unwanted pregnancy and to guard against the spread of STDs. If you have been having unprotected heterosexual intercourse and an unplanned pregnancy has been avoided thus far, you may have begun to think you're infertile. Don't keep testing this idea because, in all likelihood, you are not really sterile - you have simply been very lucky.

A doubly painful ordeal

Mary was an 18-year-old girl who was sent to me because she had behavior problems. She and her parents were having frequent arguments over setting limits and issues of independence. She did not feel that she was given enough freedom and was upset that her friends had much later curfews than she did.

I met with Mary and her parents several times to try and discover any hidden, underlying problems. Supportive counseling and simple suggestions to help relieve the tension were given. The situation at home gradually improved to the point that everyone seemed to be back on the same page. We all agreed that it was no longer necessary to keep meeting, and I returned Mary to the care of her regular doctor.

Several months later Mary returned to the office. As it turned out, the behavior difficulties seemed to have been the least of her problems. She sobbed in the exam room while she told me how she had been raped one month earlier, and now she was worried that she might be pregnant. Immediately after the rape she had been examined in an emergency room at another hospital. She was treated for her injuries and given medication to reduce the risk of contracting a sexually transmitted disease. But unfortunately, the doctor on duty did not offer her emergency birth control.

We gave Mary a pregnancy test, and it was positive. She then had to deal with an unwanted pregnancy in addition to the severe emotional damage caused by the rape. Emergency birth control works well most of the time if it is prescribed quickly, preferably within 72 hours of an unexpected exposure. Close medical supervision and follow-up are extremely important in such situations. I don't know if Mary would have chosen this medication if she had been given the opportunity in the emergency room. I do know that she had difficulty coping with the pregnancy and struggled with the decision to have to an abortion.

She finally did decide to have the abortion, and I kept a close watch on her for several months after this procedure was performed. She was a tough kid with a great deal of inner strength, which helped her get through this tender time in her life. Her parents were also very supportive and they both rallied behind their daughter.

The overall outcome was as good as could be expected under the circumstances. It could have been even better if emergency birth control had been correctly prescribed to reduce the risk of pregnancy in the first place.

★★★★★★

There needs to be greater public awareness about the availability of emergency birth control as an important preventive strategy to reduce the risk of pregnancy in the event of a rape or other unexpected sexual encounter. Young men as well as young women who are having heterosexual intercourse should be reminded that this method can be used in cases when condoms leak, slip, or break. Emergency birth control is also useful when girls who are taking oral contraceptives miss more than two birth control pills in a row, or when those who are receiving injected contraceptives every three months go more than 14 weeks after their last shot. It can also be used when types of barrier protection like diaphragms or cervical caps are dislodged or move out of position.

PARENT TIP - Think of emergency birth control as a second chance to prevent an unintended pregnancy. Be sure to include discussions on this important method when you talk to your adolescent about contraception.

While there may be no such thing as safe sex, a healthy romance can still go on without taking unnecessary risks. Prevention of STDs must continue to be a top priority at this stage. Heterosexual transmission of the human immunodeficiency virus is now the main way that teenagers get HIV in the United States. Latex condoms are the best way, besides not having sex at all, to prevent the spread of this virus and other STDs. Being involved with just one partner (monogamy) is getting more popular with older adolescents. Unfortunately, people often have a series of these one-on-one encounters, and adequate protection is frequently not used.

It is quite obvious that many vulnerable individuals are still unable to grasp the idea of disease prevention, and not even the fear of being infected with HIV has made them change their high-risk habits. The close relationship between sexual activity and other psychosocial issues of adolescence such as low self-esteem, depression, problems with friends or family, substance abuse, and so forth, needs to be emphasized. For example, young adults with body image problems may act-out sexually to get more attention. Those who are unhappy may seek comfort in close physical contact. Adolescents who have been abused may have a strong need for someone to care for them or to love them. Those who are having problems with peers or at home may look for closer, more intimate personal relationships to relieve stress and anxiety. In addition, those whose judgement is weakened by chemicals are at a very high risk for unplanned pregnancies and STDs, including HIV.

As they come down through the clouds during the final stage of adolescence, gay and lesbian youth will usually have a clearer picture of their sexual identity. Some may accept their orientation and come out to friends and family. Others may prefer to stay in the closet until they feel it is safer to let the world know where they stand. Those who continue to have unresolved conflicts and concerns about their sexual identity remain at very high risk for self-destructive behaviors such as substance abuse and suicide. This is particularly true if they do not have someone they trust, with whom they can discuss their innermost concerns. It can be a long, lonely road for those who do not have a straight orientation and who feel that there is no one to turn to for help.

CHAPTER 34

Facing Foreclosure on Life

Threats of harm to self or others may be triggered by seemingly unimportant happenings that may feel like the end of the world to adolescents. As they begin the reentry process they are better equipped to dump excess baggage and to practice proper mental hygiene. They are learning how to brush their brain and floss between the lobes to get rid of any emotional debris or decay. But as they glide downward they may still fall into unexpected pockets of turbulence with wide mood swings or periods of sadness which may tend to color their thinking. If they suddenly start singing the blues or begin to express suicidal thoughts, those close to them must listen carefully and act quickly. It should not be assumed that this is just for show, a so-called gesture or simply attention-seeking behavior. Such false thinking could prove to be a costly error, especially since teens act so impulsively. These feelings must always be taken seriously; graveyards are full of adolescents who were mistakenly mislabeled as making attention-seeking gestures. This phony diagnosis only serves to cover over the fact that these teenagers are showing signs of trouble, and it further gets in the way of proper help. The term 'gesture' should be sent to the scrap heap because it is very misleading and completely inappropriate, and may actually create yet another barrier to necessary mental health services for teens.

Feelings of sadness may gradually build up over time, or follow an important personal loss such as the death of a loved one, separation of the parents, divorce, breakup with a boyfriend or girlfriend, and so forth. Transient periods of mourning with occasional flashbacks of sadness after such happenings are normal. But sadness or mourning that continues for a long time and does not go away is not normal. Regular checkups with a mental hygienist for a quick brainstorming session or mind sweeping as needed are usually very helpful. Occasionally the services of a full-blown shrink may also be necessary.

PARENT TIP - If you decide to seek additional help for your adolescent, here are a few points to keep in mind when selecting a therapist. First, such an individual should have the proper qualifications, including sufficient training or experience with young adults. Second, the chemistry between them needs to be good so that this person will be able to connect with your son or daughter. Third, underlying medical conditions must be excluded and the correct psychiatric diagnosis must be established. Next, appropriate therapy should be started in the form of counseling as needed. Finally, the use of medication should also be carefully considered in selected situations when specifically indicated. A medical practitioner will be needed to write for any prescription drugs. By following the above sequence, you will help to assure that your adolescent gets the best care he or she deserves. Be patient, since there is an element of trial and error involved in this process. Sometimes things may not work out and you will need to find another therapist.

Ready to cash in her chips

Andrea was a 19-year-old young woman who called me one day and said that she needed to come in right away. I had seen her in consultation a couple of years earlier when she was a high school student in an outlying area. She was now attending college in my city and still had my card. She sounded very anxious on the phone so I told her to come to the office as soon as possible.

When Andrea arrived she was in pretty bad shape. I knew her fairly well from her previous visits and we had a good relationship. The once spunky girl looked almost limp as she slouched in the chair. She immediately broke down and cried. Between sobs she was able to say how unhappy she was about the way her life was going. She said that she wanted to die and didn't think she could make it through another day. She was actively suicidal and clearly had thoughts of killing herself. She felt all alone, with nowhere to go or no one to turn to. Fortunately, she was able to get up enough strength to meet with me. At that particular time I was her one and only confidant. Andrea trusted me enough to understand that as bad as she felt at that time there was no reason to believe that she would always feel that way.

I was able to convince her that there certainly was hope, but that we needed to get her additional help right away. She agreed to an immediate visit with a psychiatrist.

Andrea responded very well to antidepressant medication and outpatient therapy. She was able to stay in school and finish the semester. As I look back, I am glad she had the foresight to save my number and give me a call when she was about to hit rock bottom. It felt good to have been able to help lift her spirits and see her feeling as feisty as ever.

TEEN TIP - If you are sad, unhappy, or depressed, you don't need to go it alone. Try to contact someone you can trust and to whom you can express your innermost thoughts. Use the method of communication you are most comfortable with. This might be talking on the phone, chatting on the computer, writing a poem or a letter, sending a card, composing a song, or even making a video. The key is to communicate, whenever possible. If you continue to suffer and have no one with whom you feel you can confide, then you may need extra help. Counselors, therapists, doctors and other health professionals have been trained to help you get through the tough times. Don't be afraid to seek their advice. Remember, their only mission is to improve your health and happiness.

CHAPTER 35
Falling into Place

They're back - those teens who were able to bear the torch and survive the search for the Perfect 10. As they touch back down on Planet Earth there will be a sigh of relief from all who took part in the mission, both in the air and on the ground. Once they set foot on familiar soil, the refugees from outer space may be difficult to recognize through all the tears of joy. This is a time to roll out the red carpet and strike up the band. Family and friends who have waited patiently will be rewarded as the mature, independent, and unique individual returns at last. Even after they have landed, adolescents may still be sky high as they begin to gather their belongings, collect their faculties, and come to their senses. They may need to take a little break to catch their breath before they can figure out exactly where they stand, and finally get their act together.

As they hit the home stretch they will have traveled full circle to reach their final destination. By now they will have grown to understand that the highway to happiness is not always smooth, straight, or otherwise perfect. Sometimes they may need a little lift if they stop, stumble, or stammer along the way. Special directions may also be needed for those who are easily influenced and swayed by popular opinion, or tempted to take a short cut, or who wind up straying down a dead end street. Some parties may even enlist the services of a psychic or a fortuneteller to get an extra sense of predictability or added security. While this book may not be a crystal ball, it is envisioned that it will work more as a map, a compass, or a gyroscope so that adolescents will be able to keep their bearings and parents will not lose all their marbles.

As they widen their horizons, it is hoped that teens will learn how to use their heads first and then follow their hearts as they search to discover the treasures at the end of the rainbow. The words 'Mission Accomplished' will carry the greatest reward. If adolescents are able to live a happy, healthy life, we can all share the gold. Let's go for it!

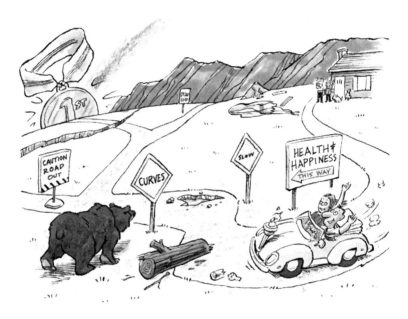

Acknowledgement

The author wishes to acknowledge Marilyn Cavanaugh, Peggy Baruch, and Diane Anderson for their review of this book, Bob Noonan for his copy-editing, and Joe Glisson for his cartoon drawings.

CPSIA information can be obtained at www.ICGtesting.com
Printed in the USA
BVOW070307080212

282415BV00002B/92/P